GETTING THE BEST OUT OF YOUR JUICER

Featuring a Comprehensive Dictionary of Juices

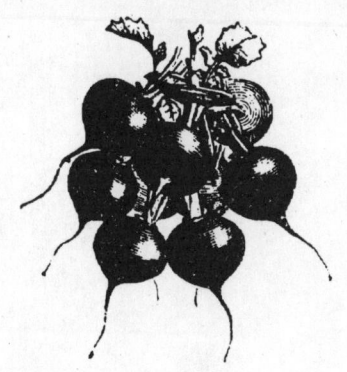

GETTING THE BEST OUT OF YOUR JUICER

William H. Lee, R.Ph., Ph.D.

Featuring a Comprehensive Dictionary of Juices

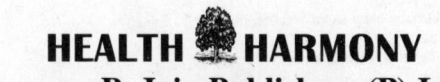
HEALTH HARMONY

An imprint of **B. Jain Publishers (P) Ltd.**
USA — EUROPE — INDIA

GETTING THE BEST OUT OF YOUR JUICER

First Edition: 2004
4th Impression: 2015

Getting the Best Out of Your Juicer is not intended as medical advice. Its intent is solely information and educational. Please consult a health professional should the need for one be indicated.

Published by Keats Publishing, Inc. 27 Pine Street (Box 876) New Canaan, Connecticut 06840-0876

© 1992 by William H. Lee

All rights reserved. No part of this book may be reproduced in any form without the written consent of the publisher.

The Appendix and portions of Chapter 2 are reproduced from the author's publication the "Hoe Do I know if I Need Vitamins and if I do which ones?" Handbook, © 1987, 1991 by William H. Lee.

Restricted to sale within Indian Subcontinent only

Published by Kuldeep Jain for

HEALTH HARMONY

An Imprint of
B. JAIN PUBLISHERS (P) LTD.
1921/10, Chuna Mandi, Paharganj, New Delhi 110 055 (INDIA)
Tel.: +91-11-4567 1000   Fax: +91-11-4567 1010
Email: info@bjain.com   Website: **www.bjain.com**

Printed in India

ISBN: 978-81-319-0195-3

Contents

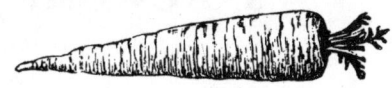

Foreword 6

1. **You & Juice** 10
   Why Homemade's Best

2. **Vitamins & Minerals** 16
   A Few Basics

3. **What's In It For You** 36
   A Dictionary of Juices
   From Alfalfa to Watermelon

4. **Index of Therapies** 90
   Juicing for Everything from
   Acne to Water Retention

5. **Juices for Cleansing** 122
   ...Juices for Healing

6. **Buying a Juicer** 128
   Your Home Juice Bar

7. **Juiced for Fun** 136
   Drinking Your Health

8. **Juice Dieting** 156
   For Easy Weight Loss

   Appendix 158
   Vitamin/Mineral Tables

Foreword

> 🌿 If I had known I was going to live this long, I'd have taken better care of myself.
>
> —Songwriter Eubie Blake, on approaching his hundredth birthday

How many times have you had the strong conviction that there was *something* you could do, some lifestyle change, that would make your life healthier and, with a little bit of luck, longer? That's probably happened fairly often, and just as often you've found that you weren't sure of it or, when you got right down to it, you weren't going to do. it. The truth is that there are any number of things we can do to make an improvement (mainly because there seem to be so many things we're doing wrong) such as exercise programs, meditation, and a huge variety of diets. And the trouble is, most of them involve a lot of effort or time or are plain boring.

There is one immense improvement you can make in your way of living, a change that is comparatively easy, quite interesting and profoundly effective—you can learn to prepare and drink substantial quantities of fresh fruit and vegetable juices.

Foreword

To answer the very natural question of what on earth fresh juices can have to do with good health and longevity, let's take a somewhat roundabout approach and start with the observation that we humans have the distinction of being the only inhabitants of this planet to cook the food we eat—most of it, in fact.

It wasn't always thus. Our remotest ancestors ate what they pulled from the ground, knocked from the trees or ran down on the plains, raw. Fruits, vegetables, wild grains and nuts formed most of their diet, with all the vitamins, minerals, enzymes and fiber intact and in the best form to nourish the eater. Neanderthal and Cro-Magnon peoples discovered and used fire, and presumably found that its action on foods softened them, made them keep longer, and added some interesting elements to their taste.

> **NOBODY NOTICED FOR SEVERAL TENS OF THOUSANDS OF YEARS THAT COOKING SEVERELY REDUCED THE NUTRITIONAL VALUE OF FOODS.**

What nobody noticed for several tens of thousands of years was that cooking also severely reduced the nutritional value of foods, leaching away minerals and vitamins in cooking water and destroying enzymes by the action of heat. Recent nutritional studies have shown this, and many others have shown that diets substantially composed of raw fruits and vegetables promote good health and longevity. A large body of verified information suggests strongly that the standard modern diet in this and other industrial countries fosters poor health—obesity and degenerative diseases in particular—and even antisocial and criminal behavior.

But there's a big gap between what studies show and what people do, between what we know makes sense and our ingrained prejudices and habits. Many people will turn to raw fruits and vegetables, and benefit from that; many more won't.

This is where fresh fruit and vegetable juices come in. They are easy to prepare, and contain an abundance of the important nutrients, particularly the living enzymes, present in the original source plants. Those who would find it hard going to get through several raw vegetables in the course of a day can get most of the benefits quickly by means of the juice, supplying their bodies with an abundance of vital nutrients and digestive factors.

Juices should not be looked at as a substitute for a sensible diet, but their use will add to the benefits of any diet. You can take them just because you enjoy their taste and want to assure yourself of a good supply of important nutrients; for that purpose we've supplied a number of good-tasting juice recipes. Or you can use them for specific therapeutic purposes, from prevention or treatment of disease to weight management; chapter 4 discusses this in detail. Preparing the juice is all-important, since if it's too messy, expensive or troublesome, you are simply not going to keep it up; chapter 8 discusses different types of juicers and their features.

All energy on Earth derives from the sun, and growing plants—fruits and vegetables—are the most available form of that energy. Fresh juices give us that energy directly and supremely pleasantly, and this book will show you why, and how to make the most of them.

FRESH FRUIT JUICES CONTAIN AN ABUNDANCE OF IMPORTANT NUTRIENTS, PARTICULARLY LIVING ENZYMES.

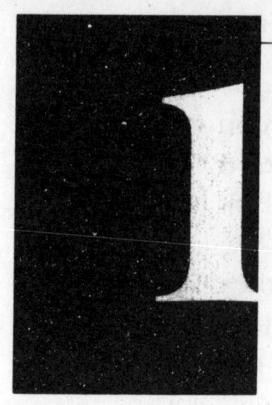

You & Juice
Why Homemade's Best

Juices are nothing new to most Americans. After mother's milk, juices are probably our first foods. Stop at the baby-food section of your supermarket and look at the variety of juices available for infants.

Or consider your own breakfast table. How often do you start your breakfast with a glass of orange or grapefruit juice, or perhaps some prune juice to keep you regular? Commercially produced bottles and cans of juices, either from natural juice or concentrate, fill shelf after shelf in most food stores.

If so many people are conscious of juices, why write a book about them or why bother to read about them?

Because there's a wide difference between the value of commercial juices and the juices you can make at home. Raw juice, prepared fresh from the fruit or vegetable, is a wonderful source of vitamins, minerals, enzymes, proteins, carbohydrates, naturally purified plant liquid, chlorophyll, and phytochemicals (natural plant chemicals which have a beneficial effect on your body).

With all of the talk and publicity being given to the value of fiber, why read a book that emphasizes extracting the juice and leaving the fiber behind?

Fiber, from fruits and vegetables and from grains, is an important part of everyone's health regimen and has to be considered when planning your daily dietary intake. Oatmeal or other cereal fiber for breakfast and raw fruit and raw or lightly seamed vegetables should be included in your diet; however, raw juices must be considered as a special category for specialized nutritional value.

It is precisely because the fiber is left behind that raw juices are the best source of nutritive value for your body! When you eat a piece of fruit it can take up to four hours for the fruit to be completely digested and the nutritional benefits distributed to the hungry cells of your body. If you eat two pieces of fruit, the bulk can prevent all of the natural goodness from being extracted and some nutritional value may be lost.

The same thing applies to your vegetable meal. Usually you may have vegetables with your lunch or dinner. You may have meat and potatoes with the vegetables, or maybe some pasta. Whatever way you're accustomed to eat, vegetables are usually a part of a meal and have to be digested along with a lot of other foods.

Figure four to six hours for complete digestion. Quite a lot of nutritional value has bypassed the system and is lost in the waste.

Now, are you ready for this? Juices are absorbed, assimilated and feeding your thirsty cells all their nutritional power in about fifteen minutes.

We're a country that thrives on quick results. We want instant gratification. So do our cells and tissues. All the nutritional value nature puts into fruits and vegetables can be available to your body only minutes after you've juiced and drunk.

JUICES ARE ABSORBED AND FEEDING YOUR THIRSTY CELLS IN ABOUT FIFTEEN MINUTES.

Then there's another thing.

You've cut up the food, put it in the juicer and made the juice. It's an honest effort and you know what you're putting in your body. Do you always know the same thing about commercially prepared juices?

🍎 One company was indicted on charges of selling millions of bottles of "apple juice" which turned out to be sugar-water. The label claimed it to be 100 percent apple juice, and it was sold for five years to unsuspecting mothers for their children.

🍎 "Florida squeezed" juices may be made from fruit that has been imported from countries that use insecticides banned in the United States. The fruit is brought in and "squeezed" in Florida, hence the label.

🍎 Concentrates can be wonderfully stocked with all the nutritional value of the fruit. Take the concentrate home and mix it with bottled water or your own sink water if it's good-tasting and you'll have a drink almost as good as if you juiced it yourself. But where did the company that pre-mixed the juice and put it in a bottle or carton get its water from?

🌶 Is the juice you've made not as pretty as the juice prepared commercially? Maybe they've added artificial color or flavor...or even chemical preservatives!

You've made a decision to enhance and protect your health. Raw juices are better for you than soft drinks, coffee, black teas, and are also better than most of the juices you see in the food store.

But there's more to the raw juice story. Raw juices may also prevent or help heal diet-related illnesses.

There's a whole new field of "neutraceuticals" coming into being. Its aim is to understand and utilize the growing array of food and nutritional products with significant health and medical benefits. The rapidly increasing knowledge of the role of various nutrients in specific diseases has scientists working on designer foods. The potential role of nutrients in disease prevention is staggering. Nutrients are being studied for such far-reaching benefits as slowing the aging process and countering the adverse health effects of pollution. University-based clinical studies published in respected medical journals show the value of an ever-broadening range of nutritional substances in the prevention and treatment of specific diseases.

NUTRIENTS ARE BEING STUDIED FOR SUCH FAR-REACHING BENEFITS AS SLOWING AGING AND COUNTERING POLLUTION.

One of the most startling examples of the growth of knowledge about the importance of nutrition and health is media acceptance. Both *Time* Magazine and *The New York Times*, traditionally wedded to conventional medical views on health and disease, gave extensive space to favorable treatments of vitamins and nutrients as health enhancers in early 1992, citing the studies showing that certain foods and supplements could prevent or reverse many of the most serious diseases. Study report topics include the use of beta-carotene to prevent lung cancer, vitamin B-6 to treat and prevent diabetic hypertension, vitamin A to treat measles, antioxidants to reduce damage from heart attacks, cabbage juice to treat ulcers, apple and prune juices to aid regularity, watermelon and cucumber juices as diuretics.

And there's still more to come.

Most people are aware that fruits and vegetables contain vitamins and minerals, but this new nutritional revolution has uncovered hitherto unknown treasures like:

• Tomato juice contains GABA—gamma-aminobutyric acid—which can lower hypertension. It also contains cancer-preventing lycopene.

• Grapefruit juice contains vitamin C and cancer-preventing limonene. The grapefruit pectins can help lower cholesterol.

🕭 Citrus juices contain flavonoids, which enhance the body's detoxification system. They also contain phenolocs, which can neutralize carcinogens.

The list of therapeutic functions of juices is steadily getting longer, but that's only a part of the story. Of course, the use of juices to help eliminate disease is a marvel. However, why not utilize juices in the prevention of disease on a regular basis? No one is claiming that drinking raw juices daily will prevent anything from happening to you, but incorporating juices in a nutritious and balanced diet, along with following an exercise program, should lead to a long and healthful life.

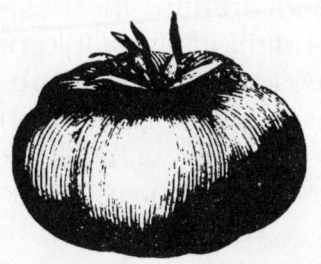

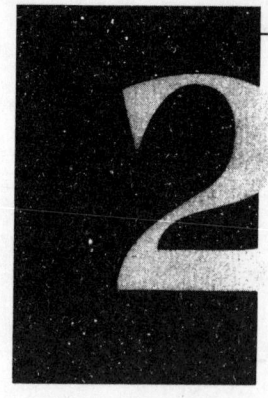

2 Vitamins & Minerals

A Few Basics

We Americans are the best-fed and the least nutritionally stable people in the world, considering that we are a first-class nation. The Standard American Diet (SAD) leaves many of us with full stomachs but nutritionally short-changed. The lack of one or more nutrients can have serious consequences to your health. The following material describes the body's uses of vitamins and minerals and the problems that may occur if there is a prolonged lack in the diet. If such a deficiency is allowed to continue, if you ignore the warning signs, you can endanger your health and well-being.

The sensible thing is to make certain that your diet is rich in the nutrients your lifestyle calls for. These nutrients are remark-

> **THE LACK OF NUTRIENTS CAN AFFECT YOUR BODY IN GROSS OR IN SUBTLE WAYS.**

ably easy to obtain through a varied diet—and the use of raw juices.

This chapter will. enable you to check your own health against the following symptoms which may be caused by nutrient shortfall. There is also a list of fruits and vegetables suitable for juicing which contain the essential vitamins and minerals to keep you on the plus side of deficiency.

The lack of nutrients in sufficient amounts can affect your body in gross or in subtle ways.

VITAMINS

We'll start with the vitamins—those substances we almost always have to get from food or supplements—and discuss their general functions in the body, following up with a list of fruits and vegetables whose juice provides abundant quantities of each vitamin. (For those interested in more detailed information, the Appendix provides a complete table of vitamins and minerals, their recommended intake, food sources, antagonists, body systems affected, and deficiency symptoms.)

Vitamin A

Although most people think of vitamin A as only for the health of the eyes, it actually benefits the entire body. Vitamin A is necessary for the continued good health of all of the mucous membrane of the mouth, ears, stomach, etc. It helps to guard against infection, and it helps to build teeth, bones and blood.

It is a stimulant to our body's defense system and helps keep our sex organs in good repair.

Vitamin A is usually obtained from either fish liver oils or vegetables. When it is taken from vegetable sources, as in juices, it is called beta-carotene. There can be an overdose of vitamin A (it happens very rarely), but there can never be a toxic overdose of beta-carotene, although really vast over-consumption of carrot juice can temporarily yellow the skin.

Vitamin B-Complex

The individual B vitamins are discussed in the Appendix. The B-complex vitamins are water-soluble and cannot be stored in the body. They must be obtained from food and from supplements every day.

The *Nutrition Almanac* states:

The B-complex vitamins are active in providing the body with energy, basically by converting carbohydrates into glucose which the body "burns" to produce energy. They are vital in the metabolism of fats and protein. In addition, the B vitamins are necessary for the normal functioning of the nervous system and may be the single most important factor for the health of nerves. They are essential for the maintenance of muscle tone in the gastrointestinal tract and for the health of the skin, hair, eyes, mouth, and liver.

THE B VITAMINS MAY BE THE SINGLE MOST IMPORTANT FACTOR FOR THE HEALTH OF THE NERVES.

This begins to give you an indication of the importance of vitamins to good health.

> *The Vitamin B-complex Family*
> thiamine (vitamin B-1)
> riboflavin (vitamin B-2)
> niacin (vitamin B-3—also known as niacinamide)
> pyridoxine (vitamin B-6)
> cyanocobalamin (vitamin B-12)
> biotin
> choline
> inositol
> folic acid
> para-aminobenzoic acid (PABA)
> pantothenic acid (calcium pantothenate)

Vitamin C
Vitamin C is the healing vitamin, the protective vitamin, the most talked-about vitamin and deservedly so. Vitamin C may be one of the best answers to pollution and promoters of longer life and healthier old age. Most animals can manufacture their own vitamin C. We can't, and since it is water-soluble, we have to have quantities of it daily. Vitamin C helps maintain the connective tissue that holds us together. It fights infections, relieves allergies, combats radioactivity, fights cancer and the common cold. It is one of the greatest supplements we can find.

Vitamin D
Also known as "the sunshine vitamin." One of the first questions a nutritionist will be asked during a lecture is "Why must

WE CAN MAKE VITAMIN D OURSELVES, BUT WE'D HAVE TO RUN AROUND NAKED FOR MOST OF THE DAY.

we take vitamin D as a supplement when we can manufacture it in our own body?"

It's true! We can make vitamin D ourselves, but we'd have to run around naked for most of the day. There could not be any smog to deflect the sun's rays, and when oil formed on our skin, which contained vitamin D, we'd have to wait for it to be absorbed and not jump into the pool or into a shower. Now you see why it is recommended as a supplement. Without it, calcium and phosphorus for strong bones and teeth cannot be absorbed!

Vitamin E
The antioxidant action of vitamin E helps to prevent the breakdown of fatty substances in the body, keeping the body healthier, and perhaps younger. Vitamin E helps to increase the flow of blood to the heart, helps promote healing inside and outside, and helps stimulate the reproductive organs to prevent miscarriages.

According to the Vitamin Nutrition Information Service, these are the vitamins people most commonly take:
- multi-vitamins
- B vitamins
- vitamin E
- vitamin C
- vitamins A & D

Nearly 60 million adults take vitamins every day.

Individual vitamins are more often used when people have symptoms that they believe will respond to vitamin therapy. Vitamin users tend to believe in prevention more than they believe in treatment. Juice therapy is emerging as one of the most effective ways to assure ourselves of a healthful abundance of vitamins. And the same is true of minerals.

MINERALS

Minerals are the unsung heroes of the nutritional field. The balance of quantities in the body is delicate and vital. Mineral deficiencies are becoming more frequent as the amounts of minerals in the soil is depleted. If it's not in the soil then it can't be in the food.

There are six essential minerals: calcium, phosphorus, iodine, iron, zinc and magnesium; and a number of trace minerals necessary for human health (copper, chromium, manganese, molybdenum, selenium, sodium, potassium. etc.). There are also other trace minerals which have some bearing on human nutrition but our explorations have not yet determined the specific part they play (lithium, silver, nickel, barium, boron, etc.)

Calcium
One of the body's most abundant minerals. It is found primarily in the bones and teeth. It works with phosphorus, magnesium, vitamin A, and vitamin C to build bones. It aids cardiovascular health, relates to muscle growth and muscle movement (is often used to help relieve menstrual cramps along with magnesium, vitamin B-6, vitamin E), can act as a natural sedative when taken at night.

There are various supplements that can be purchased, and it is best to take them in divided doses throughout the day,. Some may be mixtures of calcium and vitamin D to insure absorption. Calcium ascorbate is a combination of calcium and vitamin C while a preparation of calcium orotate is a mixture of calcium and orotic acid. Different people benefit differently from supplements derived from various sources.

Magnesium

As mentioned, it works with calcium. It also is involved in regulating blood sugar levels and cholesterol metabolism and is helpful in heart conditions.

Calcium supplements include magnesium for the most part. Nutritionists recommend the use of twice as much calcium as magnesium.

Iron

Iron and calcium are the two minerals found to be most deficient in the diets of American women. This is very unfortunate since calcium is necessary to prevent osteoporosis (bone decay) and iron is important for building strong, red blood. Good blood promotes resistance to disease and to stress. It also provides good transportation for oxygen all over the body. Iron requires vitamin C to be absorbed from the intestinal tract.

Zinc

A lack of zinc can cause a depressive state. It aids in maintaining blood sugar levels, digesting food, resisting viral infections and preventing acne. It helps wounds to heal (they may not heal without it). Zinc and pumpkin seed oil have often been used to help soothe prostate troubles. Although many compounds of zinc have been shown to be helpful, new research done with zinc picolinate substantiates the effectiveness of this new zinc complex.

Selenium
Increases resistance to infection, disease and free radicals. Works very well with vitamin E to protect cell membrane. It may help to prevent hardening of tissues and stave off the aging process.

Since this is merely a glance at all of the nutritional factors that go into good health, I'd like to suggest that you read as much as you can about all of the vitamins and minerals. Knowledge can keep you healthy.

TRACE MINERALS

Trace minerals are elements that occur in the body in very minute amounts. Though their presence within the body, is small, in most cases, they have been shown to be necessary for health.

Potassium
It is found mainly inside the cell walls while its partner, sodium, is found mainly outside the cell walls. These two minerals work together to form what is termed the sodium/potassium "pump." They help regu-

late water balance within the body—which means regulating the distribution of fluids on either side of the cell walls and moving nutrients in and out of the cells. Potassium works to control the activity of heart muscles, nervous system and kidneys. It is important as an alkalizing agent in keeping proper acid-alkaline balance in the blood and tissues. It prevents overacidity. It promotes secretion of hormones.

Iodine

It is essential for the health of the thyroid gland and for the formation of thryroxin (the thyroid hormone which regulates much of physical and mental activity). Iodine regulates the rate of metabolism, energy production, and body weight. It helps prevent rough and wrinkled skin caused by a deficiency.

Manganese

It is an important component of several enzymes which are involved in metabolism of carbohydrates, fats and proteins. Combined with choline (a B vitamin), it helps in fat digestion and utilization. It helps to nourish the nerves and brain. It is involved in the function of the reproductive organs and the mammary glands.

Phosphorus

It works with calcium to build bones and teeth. It is important in the utilization of carbohydrates, fats and proteins for the growth, maintenance and repair of cells and also for the production of energy. It is needed for healthy nerves and for efficient mental activity. It is an important factor in maintaining an acid/alkaline balance in the blood and tissues.

Chloride
Bonded with sodium or potassium. it is essential for the production of hydrochloric acid in the stomach. which is needed for proper protein digestion and for mineral assimilation. It helps to maintain joints and tendons. It helps the liver in its detoxifying activity. It is involved in the maintenance of proper fluid and electrolyte balance in the system.

Sulphur
It is vital for healthy hair, skin and nails. It is necessary for collagen synthesis. It is essential for the formation of body tissues. It plays a part in tissue respiration. It works with the liver to secrete bile. It also helps to maintain overall body balance.

Copper
It aids in the formation of red blood cells, It is part of many enzymes. It works with vitamin C to form elastin. It is necessary for the production of RNA. It is involved in protein metabolism, in healing processes, and in keeping the natural color of the hair. It aids in the development of bones, brain, nerves and connective tissues.

Fluoride
It is essential for bone and tooth building. It protects against infections.

Chromium
It is an integral part of many enzymes and hormones. It is a cofactor with insulin to remove glucose from the blood into the cells. It is essential for proper utilization of sugar. It stimulates the activity of enzymes involved in the metatabolism of energy and synthesis of fatty acids, cholesterol and protein. Look for GTF chromium in your supplement. It is chromium, niacin, glycine, glutamic acid and cysteine in the trivalent form, the form most easily utilized by the body.

Cobalt
It functions as part of vitamin B 12. It maintains red blood cells. It activates a number of enzymes in the body.

Molybdenum
It is a component of several important enzymes and a catalyst for some unique chemical reactions in the body.

THE WONDERFUL WORLD OF AMINO ACIDS

Next to water, protein is the most plentiful substance in the body. One-third is found in muscles and the rest in bones, skin, cartilage, blood and other body substances. Protein transports nutrients in and out of cells and is responsible for their growth, maintenance and regeneration. Protein is also needed for the formation of hormones and enzymes. It is important to the immune system, as it is used to make antibodies and white blood cells.

All protein is made up of amino acids. They are the "building blocks" of life. The amino acids join together in an infinite variety of ways to form the various different kinds of proteins. There are approximately 22 different kinds of amino acids. Some can be made in the body and are termed "nonessential." There are eight that cannot be produced in the body and they are considered the "essential" amino acids. Children have ten essential aminos. These must be supplied by the diet or as food supplements. When all the essential amino acids are found in a food in relatively equal amounts, that food is called a *complete protein*. Foods that lack or are extremely low in one or more of the essential amino acids are called *incomplete proteins*. Meats, fish, poultry and dairy products are complete protein foods. Most vegetables, grains and fruits are incomplete protein foods. Incomplete protein foods can be combined to obtain a balance of all the essential aminos and thereby provide a complete protein meal.

The eight essential acids are lysine, methionine, leucine, threonine, valine. tryptophan, isoleucine, and phenylalanine. In addition, histidine and arginine are considered essential for children to support growth.

WHICH JUICES HAVE WHAT VITAMINS AND MINERALS AND AMINO ACIDS?

Nutrient	Raw Juice Source
Vitamin A	Carrots, spinach, tomatoes, red and green peppers, cabbage, celery, rose hips, citrus fruits
Vitamin B1	Grapefruit, carrots, beets, beet tops, celery, green peppers, spinach, dandelion, pineapple, asparagus
Vitamin B2	Parsley, turnip greens, broccoli, asparagus, carrots, beet tops, celery, green peppers, kale, spinach
Vitamin B3	Parsley, kale, potatoes, asparagus
Vitamin B5	Cabbage, cauliflower, strawberries, grapefruit, oranges
Vitamin B6	Pears, spinach, lemons, potatoes, carrots
Folic acid	Spinach, parsley, carrots, potatoes, oranges, asparagus, broccoli, Brussels sprouts
Biotin	Cauliflower, spinach, lettuce, grapefruit
Inositol	Oranges, grapefruit, cabbage, cauliflower, kale, beets, tomatoes, onions
Vitamin C	Citrus fruits, black currants, green peppers, kale, cabbage, spinach, parsley, strawberries, cantaloupes, broccoli, tomatoes

Nutrient	Raw Juice Source
Vitamin K	Spinach cabbage, carrot tops
Vitamin E	Cabbage, leeks, sprouts, green leafy vegetables
Bioflavonoids	Citrus fruits, black currants
Choline	Green leafy vegetables
PABA (para-aminobenzoic acid)	Asparagus, broccoli, green leafy vegetables, Brussels sprouts
Chlorophyll	Deep green vegetables, lettuce, kale, collard greens, chard, alfalfa sprouts, cabbage, spinach, turnip greens, watercress, parsley, celery, green peppers
Calcium	Lemons, tangerines, elderberries, kale, mustard greens, carrots, kohlrabi, watercress, cabbage, turnip tops, beet tops
Potassium	Grapes, tangerines, lemons, parsley, spinach, potatoes, dandelions, celery, kale
Sodium	Cherries, peaches, beets, kale, carrots, celery, tomatoes
Magnesium	Elderberries, raspberries, lemons, endive, beets

Nutrient	Raw Juice Source
Phosphorus	Grapes, raspberries, tangerine, spinach, carrots, cabbage, bean tops, watercress, kale
Sulphur	Black currants, red currants, spinach, watercress
Iron	Asparagus, cherries, apricots, raspberries, prunes, red currants, black currants, spinach, parsley, beet tops
Copper	Black currants, red currants, kale, potatoes, asparagus
Manganese	Strawberries, apricots, oranges, green lettuce, spinach, kale, apples, pineapple
Zinc	Apples, pears, kale, carrots, lettuce, asparagus
Cobalt	Apples, tomatoes, cabbage, carrots, beet tops, potatoes, yellow onions
Fluorine	Black currants, cherries, carrots, spinach
Iodine	Oranges, spinach
Silicon	Strawberries, grapes, lettuce, string beans, carrots
Chromium	Bananas, blueberries, oranges, strawberries, cabbage, peppers (bell and sweet), potatoes, spinach
Selenium	Garlic

Essential Amino Acids

As you glance over the sources of amino acids from the plant world you will find no strangers. At one time or another most of them were used as medicines. People versed in tribal lore would gather them and use the proper food when a particular set of symptoms was observed, much in the same manner as herbs were used. There was no distinction between herbs, foods and medicines.

The new medicine declares that you should use these foods before any symptoms are observed, thereby preventing the illness in the first place. Makes a lot more sense. What diet causes, diet can prevent.

> FOR PEOPLE VERSED IN TRIBAL LORE, THERE WAS NO DISTINCTION BETWEEN HERBS, FOODS AND MEDICINES.

Although many foods are repeated in the lists of protein suppliers, the variety of foods displayed reinforces the concept of drinking a variety of fruits and vegetables in order to give your body all of the nutrients needed.

Nutrient	Raw Juice Source
Histidine	Apple, pineapple, pomegranate, papaya, horseradish, radish, carrot, beet, celery, cucumber, endive, leek, garlic, onion, dandelion greens, turnip greens, alfalfa, spinach, sorrel

Nutrient	Raw Juice Source
Arginine	Alfalfa, carrot, beet, cucumber, celery, lettuce, leek, radish, potato, parsnip
Leucine and isoleucine	Papaya, avocado, olive
Lysine	Papaya, apple, apricot, pear, grapes, carrot, beet, cucumber, celery, parsley
Methionine	Pineapple, apple, watermelon, Brussels sprouts, cabbage, cauliflower, horseradish, chives, garlic
Phenylalanine	Pineapple, apple, carrot, beet, spinach, parsley, tomato
Threonine	Papaya, carrot, alfalfa, green leafy vegetables
Tryptophan	Carrot, beet, celery, endive, dandelion, greens, fennel, snap beans, Brussels sprouts, chives, spinach, alfalfa
Valine	Apple, pomegranate, carrot, turnip, lettuce, parsnip, squash, celery, beet, parsley, okra, tomato

ENZYMES AND CHLOROPHYLL

We are all aware of vitamins, minerals, proteins and carbohydrates; however, none of them can do any work in your body without enzymes!

Enzymes are complex biochemical substances which regulate and govern the behavior and function of all living matter. Every biochemical action that takes place in nature is caused by a specific enzyme. Fruit ripening, seeds sprouting, trees growing, people digesting food are examples of enzyme activity.

Muscle movement, sight, hearing, breathing are also examples of enzyme activity. Without enzymes, life itself would be impossible.

Why is this important to raw juice therapy?

Canned orange juice looks and tastes like fresh orange juice. The canned orange juice has no enzymes but fresh juice has. Pasteurized milk and fresh, raw milk are similar in color and taste but pasteurized milk contains no enzymes.

VITAMINS, MINERALS, PROTEINS AND CARBOHYDRATES CAN'T WORK WITHOUT ENZYMES.

Enzymes cannot stand heat.

Whenever food is cooked or boiled (212 degrees) the enzymes contained in that food are completely destroyed.

Raw juices bring all of their enzymes along with them.

The first stages of food digestion are performed by the enzymes present in the food itself. As the fruit or vegetable is juiced, the enzymes present are released in the same manner as would happen if the fruit or vegetable were chewed. The enzymes then begin the digestion process so the body has to supply very little energy to complete the digestive process and release the nutrients into the bloodstream for distribution throughout the body.

The ability to obtain natural nutrients in so easy a manner can be especially important for us as we grow older. As we age, the body's ability to manufacture enzymes slows down. Enzyme content in the body decreases with age and with disease. When you eat cooked food, the body has to supply all the enzymes for the digestive process. This costs the body energy that it could use for other purposes.

> CHLOROPHYLL IS EFFECTIVE AS AN INTERNAL ANTISEPTIC, CELL STIMULATOR, RED BLOOD BUILDER, AND REJUVENATOR.

Therefore, it would be a good idea to consume at least 30 percent of your diet in the natural state when in optimal health, including fresh, raw juices—and even more raw juices when in a less than optimal state of health.

Athletes would serve their bodies better by utilizing raw fruit and vegetable juices to replenish lost fluid than by using the commercial preparations which contain a lot of sucrose.

Raw fruits and vegetables are also wonderful sources of chlorophyll. Chlorophyll is nature's healer and cleanser. It is effective as an internal antiseptic, cell stimulator. red blood builder, and rejuvenator. The chlorophyll molecule is remarkably similar to hemoglobin, the substance that carries oxygen in the blood. The basic difference is that hemoglobin contains iron in the center of its molecule while chlorophyll contains magnesium. It's strange that red blood looks green under ultraviolet light while green chlorophyll appears to be red! Although there are chlorophyll products available in health food stores, obtaining it from raw fresh juices will make you healthier and able to fight off diseases more easily.

The best juice sources of chlorophyll are lettuce, kale, collard greens, swiss chard, alfalfa, cabbage, spinach, turnip greens, watercress, parsley, celery, cucumber, green pepper, scallions. However, any leafy greens in season will supply nature's own green medicine.

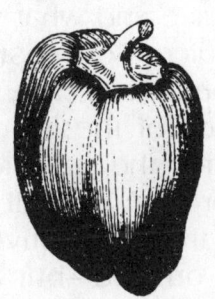

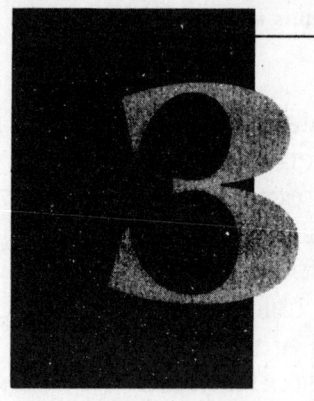

3 What's In It For You

A Dictionary of Juices from Alfalfa to Watermelon

Here's the heart of this book—a comprehensive list (A to W, anyhow, which is pretty comprehensive) of fruits and vegetables you can juice and what you can expect to find in the juice. For most, we provide a list of "natural benefits," briefly highlighting the therapeutic uses of the juiced fruit or vegetable. For some, the specific health effects are not very precise or well known, or are made clear in the descriptive text, and the benefits list is omitted—but all fresh juices provide healthful, enjoyable nourishment, and should be taken for pleasure at least as much as to remedy or prevent illness.

Alfalfa

All health food stores carry alfalfa tablets but the nutritional value of this vegetable is best obtained by juicing alfalfa sprouts. Many people consider alfalfa among the most nutritive plants on Earth. Its roots can reach thirty or forty feet into the subsoilcrawing in the minerals that have been lying fallow in virgin soil.

Alfalfa juice contains appreciable amounts of the following, as well as trace minerals: calcium, chlorine, magnesium, phosphorus, potassium, silicon, sodium, zinc.

> **ALFALFA'S ROOTS CAN REACH FORTY FEET INTO THE SUBSOIL, DRAWING IN BURIED MINERALS.**

Alfalfa sprout juice also contains a full range of vitamins: A, B-complex, C, E and K.

The juice is also a splendid source of chlorophyll and amino acids.

Buy fresh alfalfa sprouts in your health food store or grow them for yourself. The juice blends well with all other juices and can be used on a daily basis.

Apple

Rich in iron, silicon, magnesium, chlorine, copper, manganese, phosphorus, potassium, sodium and sutphur. The mineral content makes apple juice especially useful to hair, skin and nails.

Natural Benefits
- stimulates muscles and nerves
- helps eliminate uric acid
- pectin content helps reduce cholesterol
- promotes normal digestion
- promotes normal liver function
- has laxative properties

Its vitamin content is superior, with large amounts of A, B-complex, C, biotin, folic acid.

It's rich in malic acid, which is both cleansing and healing in cases of inflammation.

If possible, obtain unwaxed apples so you can wash the skin and use it as well as the pulp. Organic apples are the best for this purpose because a lot of the nutrition is in the skin as is the fruit pectin which is so helpful for peristalsis. Look for Cortland, Granny Smith, McIntosh, Golden Delicious and Pippin apples, since they are all good juicers. Select hard, crisp apples instead of the mushier ones.

> ORGANIC APPLES ARE THE BEST, BECAUSE A LOT OF THE NUTRITION IS IN THE SKIN.

Apricot

This golden fruit contains a load of vitamin C whether it is unripe or ripe, but the beta-carotene content (provitamin A) is greatest when it is fully ripened. There is twice as much vitamin A in the ripe fruit.

Natural Benefits
- builds healthy muscle and nerve tissue
- stimulates the appetite
- can have a laxative action
- is astringent to the stomach
- may be beneficial in treating anemia
- stimulating when applied to normal facial skin, and promotes healthy skin tone
- 100 grams of apricot supplies 45 percent of the normal daily requirements of vitamin A

It is also a source of vitamin B-complex and minerals, including magnesium, phosphorus, iron, calcium, potassium, sodium, suphur, manganese, cobalt and bromine.

Jerusalem Artichoke (Sunchoke)

The Jerusalem artichoke is like a potato wearing a thistle hat. Surprisingly, it makes a great juice. This vegetable is very rich in phosphorus and iron and loaded with natural inulin, which is hydrolized to levulose by the stomach acids to produce natural energy. It is this property that caused Edgar Cayce, among other natural food people, to recommend it for diabetics, hypoglycemics, and for those in need of weight reduction.

> EDGAR CAYCE RECOMMENDED THE JERUSALEM ARTICHOKE FOR DIABETICS, HYPOGLYCEMICS, AND THOSE IN NEED OF WEIGHT REDUCTION.

> Natural Benefits
> - helps diabetics
> - controls hypoglycemia
> - aids weak stomach
> - provides energy
> - enhances lactation
> - fights infection
> - diet aid

Mix 2 ounces of artichoke juice with 6 ounces of carrot for good effect.

Artichoke (Globe)

The "real" artichoke is rich in vitamins A and B-complex, and in minerals such as manganese, phosphorus and iron. It also contains inulin (not insulin), which can be used as an energy source similar to sugar, but does not require the action of the body's

> *Natural Benefits*
> - provides energy
> - stimulates the appetite
> - increases bile flow from the liver
> - stimulates circulation
> - promotes diuresis
> - combats toxins
> - aids elimination of urea, cholesterol and uric acid

insulin to be utilized. This can be a boon to diabetics, since it provides energy without taxing their insulin store.

Asparagus

You will find this vegetable in the white or green variety. The white may be grown underground and harvested as soon as the tips break ground. The green has a greater vitamin content because the sunshine has nourished it green. Either variety is cleansing to the body, and clever people buy large amounts when it is in season. They cut off the tops and steam them for a delightful meal but juice the tough stems for their mineral and other nutrient content.

ASPARAGUS IS A WONDERFUL DIURETIC AND COMPLETELY SAFE WHEN MENSTRUATION CAUSES WATER RETENTION

Asparagus is highly alkaline. It contains asparagine, which helps to cleanse the blood and body of waste material. Asparagine passes quickly through the body and imparts an odor similar to cat pee to your urine. Don't worry about it, it only means your juice is working the way it should.

> *Natural Benefits*
> - promotes normal bowel function
> - enhances action of kidneys; liver and intestines
> - helps rejuvenate skin cells
> - helpful for:
>   anemia
>   eye problems
>   nervous disorders

Asparagus is a wonderful diuretic and completely safe when menstruation causes water retention. It also is a prime source of rutin, one of the bioflavonoids that help keep capillaries flexible and in good shape.

It contains large amounts of vitamin A, C and B-complex as well as potassium, manganese and iron

Bean Sprouts

Lentils, mung beans and Aduki beans make for good sprouting. They make an excellent source of protein. Bean sprouts provide iron and vitamin C. The combination makes for better than usual iron absorption. Bean sprout juice mixes well with other vegetable juices.

BEAN SPROUTS PROVIDE IRON AND VITAMIN C, MAKING FOR BETTER THAN USUAL IRON ABSORPTION.

> *Natural Benefits*
> - blood builder
> - fatigue relief
> - controls fluid retention
> - promotes circulation
> - can relieve muscular weakness

Beans (green, string, yellow)

Green, string and yellow beans should be crisp, long and slender, and full of juice. Beans provide good quantities of vitamin A, B complex, calcium and potassium. Green beans have a higher level of vitamin A than the other varieties but the same levels of all other nutrients. One advantage of juicing is that you don't have to snip off the stems. Use the stem, peel, leaves and seeds, and juice away. Half a glass daily, mixed with carrot juice can be a therapeutic dose.

Natural Benefits
- promotes normal activity of liver and pancreas
- helps relieve rheumatism and gout
- useful for fatigue caused by overwork
- helpful for:

    anemia   diabetes
    hypoglycemia   skin problems
    thyroid problems overweight

Green beans contain inositol (found in the strings) with the rest of the B-complex, and few vegetables supply as much.

Beets

"Eat your beets, they're good for you." Beets are good because both the roots and the leafy top are edible and highly nutritious. Look for firm, smooth roots with no signs of worm damage. Old beets (like some old people) are wrinkled and flabby. If the beet is too large it will be woody and have a thick skin. Beets with round bottoms are reported sweeter than flat-bottomed ones. Tops should be fresh, vibrant, and crisp. Avoid tough, wilted or slimy beet greens with yellow leaves.

BEET TOPS CONTAIN MORE IRON THAN SPINACH.

Beets are good blood builders and body cleanser. The tops are loaded with chlorophyll and both tops and root are fine sources of vitamins A, C and B6. The tops contain more iron than spinach and top and root contain an abundance of calcium, potassium, choline, organic sodium and natural sugars. Beets are also a source of amino acids.

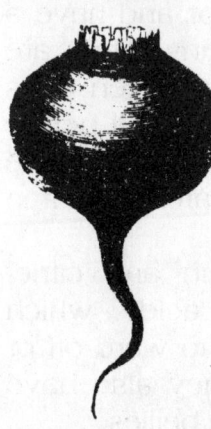

Natural Benefits
- highly nutritious
- appetite stimulant
- easily digested
- helpful for:

anemia	bladder problems
anxiety	circulatory weakness
neuritis	low blood pressure
fatigue	menstrual problems
jaundice	menopausal problems
skin problems	high blood pressure
liver problems	kidney problems

Beet juice is too powerful to take in large amounts. It's best to mix one or two ounces with carrot juice. If you prefer, the juice also mixes well with apple or cucumber.

Blackberry

Blackberries and raspberries are close relatives. Both grow on thorny brambles and have distinct fruit shapes. A single berry is actually a group of "droplets," tiny fruits clustered together. Each droplet contains a seed.

Blackberries contain vitamins A and C

> *Natural Benefits*
> - astringent
> - nutritive
> - relieves diarrhea

and some minerals as well as malic acid and isocitric acid. The acids make them astringent and valuable for diarrhea.

Blueberry

Call them whortleberry, bilberry, hurtleberry, but they're still blueberries. Ripe, fresh blueberries are plump, full of color and have a powdery "bloom" on their skins. They are highly perishable, lasting only seven days after picking, so examine them well before you buy. Dark, soft or shiny berries or those in stained or leaky containers are best left in the store.

The berries contain tannin and citric, malic, tartaric, and benzoic acids, which helps account for their ability to ward off or control bladder problems. They also have loads of vitamin C in their blue bellies.

Blueberry leaves help lower blood sugar when taken as juice by diabetics.

Myrtillin, the coloring matter of blueberries, combats colon bacillus and other germs.

> *Natural Benefits*
> - astringent to help combat infections
> - dissolves uric acid
> - protects blood vessel walls
> - combats arteriosclerosis
> - improves night vision
> - helps treat diarrhea
> - helpful against canker sores

Broccoli

Broccoli is said to be the original cauliflower and belongs to the cabbage family. Crisp, fresh, and green broccoli is most nutritious. Good supplies of vitamins A, B, C as well as potassium, sodium, iron, phosphorus, calcium, B-complex and protein.

> NEW RESEARCH APPEARS TO HAVE ISOLATED THE CANCER-FIGHTING SUBSTANCE IN CRUCIFEROUS VEGETABLES, PRESENT IN GREATEST ABUNDANCE IN BROCCOLI.

Broccoli is one of the cruciferous vegetables doctors now recommend as cancer-fighters. New research, reported in *The New York Times* in March 1992, appears to have isolated the cancer-fighting substance in cruciferous vegetables, a chemical called sulforaphane, and to show that it is present in greatest abundance in broccoli.

Brussels sprouts

This new member of the cabbage family, only 400 years old, looks like a miniature cabbage and is one of the best sources of vitamin C and beta-carotene when it is taken uncooked. Cooked Brussels sprouts lose half of their nutritive value. A combination of Brussels sprout juice, carrot juice, and lettuce juice improves the insulin-producing capacity of the pancreas. That's good news for diabetics.

Cabbage

Cabbage is the people's food. It is the "cole" in coleslaw. Cole is an archaic English term used for plants in the Brassica family, which includes broccoli, Brussels sprouts, cauliflower, kale and kohlrabi. Bok choy is the Chinese variety, and is also loaded with good nutrients. When buying, avoid cabbage with thin, wilted leaves, puffy or cracked heads, pale color or signs of insect damage. It's a good source of fiber, vitamins A, C and B-complex, potassium, magnesium and calcium. It is also a member of the cancer-fighters club.

Natural Benefits
- helpful for:

  bladder problems bronchitis
  colitis   constipation
  ulcers   skin problems
  kidney problems   asthma
  high blood pressure

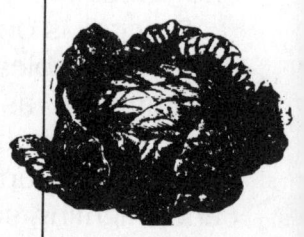

Cabbage juice is an effective laxative and skin food. Scientists agree that it has been shown to improve stomach ulcers. The sulphur content (it's the cause of the odor when cooking and the gas in your stomach) is very helpful for healing the skin and removing toxins from the body.

Mix cabbage juice with carrot juice and add a few drops of lemon juice to improve the flavor.

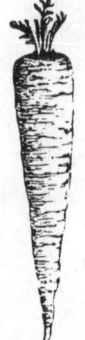

Carrots

Carrots belong to family with about 2,500 members, including parsley, parsnips, caraway, and celery. Look for smooth, firm carrots that have no cracks, bruises, soft spots or knobs. The deeper orange they are, the sweeter they are. Carrots are one of our best sources of beta-carotene, which the body

> *Natural Benefits*
> - helpful for cases of:
> | | |
> |---|---|
> | acne | arthritis |
> | asthma | bladder problems |
> | cancer | cataracts |
> | eye problems | liver problems |
> | skin problems | ulcers |
> | muscular weakness | |

converts into vitamin A. They also contain vitamins B, C, D, E and K, as well as calcium, phosphorus, potassium, organic sodium and trace minerals. The skin, hair and nails benefit greatly from carrot juice but don't get hooked on it so that you drink more than two pints a day. Your skin can take on an orange glow. Of course, it will go away as soon as you begin to cut down on the amount.

Fresh carrot juice stimulates the digestion and helps your body get rid of excess water. It also has a tonic effect on the liver and aids in cleansing this valuable organ.

CARROTS ARE ONE OF THE BEST SOURCES OF BETA-CAROTENE, WHICH THE BODY CONVERTS INTO VITAMIN A.

Celery

The greener, the more nutritious. The Pascal variety is very green, with thick ribs. The lighter celery has less nutritive value because it has been kept away from the sun. Vitamin A is found in the green leaves, while vitamin C and the B-complex are in the stems. The stalks also contain calcium, potassium, sulphur, magnesium, iron and sodium. Nutrients within the crude fibers are released during juicing and act to produce bulk, aiding in regularity.

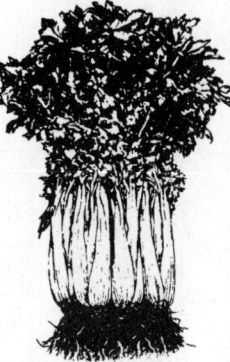

Natural Benefits
- stimulates appetite
- provides energy
- stimulates the adrenal glands
- promotes normal kidney function
- useful in:
bronchitis	nervous disorders
gout	fluid retention
constipation	insomnia

Its mineral content makes celery a good nerve tonic, nervine, and stimulant, and helps normalize body temperature during the summer's heat. Celery juice tastes salty and adds flavor to other juices when mixed together. Don't be over-cautious because of its salt content; it contains organic sodium naturally blended with other minerals and is essential to the proper functioning of the major body systems.

Chard

Often called Swiss chard, it is actually a white-rooted beet. The root is not fleshy like other beets, and it is cultivated not for the root but for the leaves, which are eaten like spinach, and the stalks, which are consumed like asparagus.

Natural Benefits
- energy builder
- laxative
- diuretic
- helpful for:
  urinary tract infections
  constipation
  skin diseases

Most chard is green, but there is a red variety now being cultivated in some areas of the United States.

Chard is a good source of vitamins A and C as well as containing quantities of iron.

Chervil

Not as well known as other vegetables but very useful, chervil contains vitamins A and C, iron and an estrogenic principle.

A juice prepared from chervil, wild cherry, lettuce and dandelion—equal parts of each—has been used as a treatment for liver and gall bladder disease.

Cherry

Cherries are related to peaches and plums. There are two main types, sweet and sour. Sweet cherries are large, heart-shaped, usually dark-colored (maroon to nearly black), and have smooth skins. The more popular varieties are Bing, Lambert, Chapman and Royal Ann. The latter variety is yellow and is typically canned, dyed red and sold as maraschino cherries.

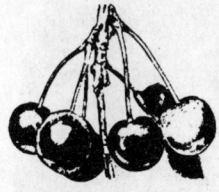

Natural Benefits
- provides energy
- promotes natural elimination
- enhances digestion
- stimulates the bile

Sour or tart cherries are smaller, round, and usually red or pinkish. Get ripe, sweet cherries that are plump, soft but not mushy. Avoid bruised, shriveled, moldy, and dull-skinned cherries.

Cherries contain vitamins A, B-complex and C as well as calcium, phosphorus, chlorine, sulphur, magnesium, sodium and potassium and the trace elements zinc, copper, manganese and cobalt. Fresh cherry juice is an aikalizer and very helpful in cases of arthritis and gout. Buy a cherry pitter to make it easier to remove the pits. The juice is quite strong and is best when mixed in equal parts with either apple juice or spring water.

Cucumber

What's long and green outside, white inside and has bumps?

Sure, you know it's a cucumber, but did you also know that the inside of a cucumber is 20 degrees Farenheit cooler than its outside temperature? That fact makes cucumber juice one of the best cooling juices for summer drinks.

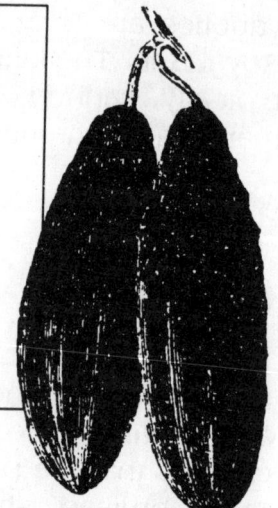

Natural Benefits
- combats toxins in the body
- energy source for muscles and nerves
- fights infection
- calms anxiety
- promotes urinary flow
- helpful adjunct in dieting
- helpful for:

  arthritis   constipation
  cramps   gout
  indigestion   rheumatism
  anemia

Look for firm cucumbers with bright-colored skins and no wrinkled or sunken spots. If the skin is waxed, you will have to remove the skin before juicing. Otherwise, juice the whole cucumber.

Cucumbers provide vitamin A, potassium, and a load of vitamin E. Cucumber juice is a natural diuretic and also promotes flexibility in the muscles and improves the elasticity of skin cells. Because it also contains silica, sulphur and trace minerals, it is important for the health of the nails and hair.

SILICA, SULPHUR AND TRACE MINERALS MAKE CUCUMBER JUICE IMPORTANT FOR THE HEALTH OF THE NAILS AND HAIR.

Currant

During the eighteenth century, black currants were considered to be a life-prolonging fruit. Currants grow like grapes in clusters and are fairly small. Currants are rich in vitamin C, protein, phosphorus, chlorine, sodium, potassium, magnesium, and calcium. Malic acid and flavonic pigments also help their nutritional profile.

Black or red currants can be juiced. You can make currant tea by mixing the juice with an equal part of hot water; it's very helpful when you have a cold.

Natural Benefits
- blood cleanser
- promotes diuresis
- eliminates uric acid
- helpful for:
  acne   fever
  skin disorders   psoriasis
  gout   cold sores
  high blood pressure

Cranberry

Another cousin of the blueberry (that's the reason cranberries and blueberries work together to help cure bladder troubles), it was named because the plant's blossoms grow downward and looks like the head of a large bird, the crane. Look for firm, bright-colored fruits. Cranberries are sorted and graded by a bounce test. They have to bounce over a barrier 4 to 7 inches in height. Those that don't pass the test are not marketed as fruit but may end up as sauce

CRANBERRY JUICE CAN BE VERY HELPFUL FOR URINARY TRACT PROBLEMS.

Cranberry juice, when taken alone, can be too acidic and sour for the average palate; it's best to mix it with apple juice. The fresh juice is rich in vitamins A, C and B complex, calcium, iron, potassium, sodium, and sulphur. If you have urinary tract problems—male or female—there is a good chance that cranberry juice will be very helpful, but not the commercial juice that has been sugared and deproved of natural enzymes. Make your own and be happy with the effect. The juice is also helpful in certain conditions when vasodilation is wanted.

Natural Benefits
- helpful for:
  asthma
  diarrhea
  fluid retention
  skin problems
  bladder problems
  fever
  indigestion

Dandelion

This can be considered to be one of nature's health tonics because it gives firmness and strength to the teeth and gums and helps prevent tooth decay. The milky juice is highly flavored and a good source of magnesium, potassium, chlorine, calcium, sulfur, iron, phosphorus, vitamins A, B-complex, and C.

> *Natural Benefits*
> - appetite stimulant
> - aids digestion
> - laxative
> - promotes diuresis
> - promotes the flow of bile
> - helps remove waste material from the body
> - Improves circulation
> - helpful for:
> | arthritis and gout | kidney problems |
> | liver problems | eye problems |

Pick the young leaves—the older ones are very bitter. Even young leaves juiced will have to be mixed with other, more pleasant-tasting juices.

Endive

This vegetable is cousin to the dandelion. When it's bright green in color, it's loaded with vitamins. Useful as a natural laxative and helpful for indigestion and liver problems. It

> *Natural Benefits*
> - helpful for:
> | bladder problems | circulation |
> | constipation | eye problems |
> | kidney problems | skin problems |

is a prime source of vitamin C as well as potassium, chlorine, calcium, sulphur, iron and phosphorus. Because it has a tangy taste, it is best mixed with carrot or celery juice.

Fennel

You may find fennel in your local store under the name finocchio. It is a relative of celery and contains an essential oil soothing to an irritated stomach. Fennel juice mixed with carrot juice is a tonic for the eyes, and, when beet juice is added to the mixture, is a tonic for the blood.

Natural Benefits
- promotes diuresis
- aids appetite
- stimulates menstrual flow
- helpful for:

skin disorders	circulation
kidney problems	liver problems
arthritis	gout

Fennel juice accompanying a meal of beans will help curb the flatulence that usually follows. It is a source of vitamins A, B-complex and C, calcium, phosphorus, sulphur, iron and potassium.

Kale

A member of the cabbage family, kale has high nutrient value when the leaves are fresh, crumpled, and have a blue-green or dark-green color. An outstanding source of vita-

29,000 units of vitamin C. Other valuable components are phosphorus, sulphur, iron, potassium and calcium, B vitamins.

The high chlorophyll content of fresh kale is another important feature of this vegetable, improving blood's ability to carry oxygen around the body. Along with endive and parsley, kale is one of the best suppliers of nutrition for the eyes. Kale's calcium content, ounce for ounce, is greater than that of milk.

> ONE GLASS OF KALE JUICE CONTAINS 27,000 UNITS OF VITAMIN A AND 29,000 UNITS OF VITAMIN C.

It's too strong-tasting to take on its own, so mix it with other green juices.

Grape

The natural blend of sugar, nutrients, and acid, bitter, mucilaginous and astringent properties make the juice acceptable to even the most delicate stomachs. In some natural

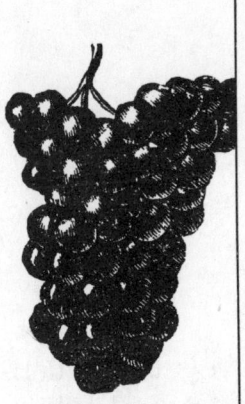

Natural Benefits
- easily digested
- superior energy supply
- loaded with vital minerals and vitamins
- stimulates normal liver function
- aids urinary flow
- enhances normal bowel function
- builds healthy skin
- juice of unripe grapes aids in clearing infections of throat and mouth
- weight loss diet adjunct
- helpful for:

cancer	gout
fever	skin probiems
rheumatism	indigestion

spas, a diet of grape juice, bread and spring water has been used to cure chronic ailments. The routine promotes the flow of urine and improves bile flow and elimination of waste material.

Grapefruit

Grapefruits contain citric acid, sugars, pectins, essential oils like limonene, pinene and citral, plus vitamins A and C, calcium, phosphorus, potassium, as well as B-complex, E, biotin, and inositol. Since the bioflavonoids are concentrated in the underskin, scrape off as much of the white part and stick it in the juicer along with the grapefruit meat. Canned juice will provide liquids during a cold, but the fresh juice will actually help combat the pain and help the body in its fight.

Natural Benefits
- aids digestion
- promotes the normal flow of urine
- weight loss diet adjunct
- helpful for:
  bruises   colds
  ear problems   fever
  indigestion   pyorrhea
  skin problems

Kohlrabi

The Germans named this vegetable "cabbage-turnip" *(kohl* = cabbage, and *rabi* = turnip) because it looks like one and tastes like the other.

> *Natural Benefits*
> - helpful for:
>   sinus problems   thyroid problems
>   skin problems   asthma

Kohlrabi can be light-skinned or purple and the smaller bulbs, about the size of a large egg, are the tastiest. The juice is good for mixing with other green juices and is a source of chlorophyll, vitamin C, iron and calcium.

Leeks

Leek juice plays internal and external roles in health. The juice mixed with milk or whey can be a soothing lotion for skin disorders of the face. It also has been used to make a poultice (mixed with bread) to be used against boils. Throat infections respond to inhalation of the steam from leeks in boiling water.

THROAT INFECTIONS RESPOND TO INHALATION OF THE STEAM FROM BOILING LEEKS.

> *Natural Benefits*
> - nerve tonic
> - promotes the flow of urine
> - laxative
> - internal antiseptic

Lettuce

Lettuce is in the same family as daisies and thistles. There are five basic types; iceberg, cos or romaine, Boston or Bibb (named after John Bibb, who developed it), leaf or lamb's lettuce, and stem—called Celtuce because it is a cross between celery and lettuce.

Romaine and Bibb are the most nutritious. The modern, cultivated lettuce is a relative of poison lettuce, a common European plant. Most lettuce is potentially narcotic and, for this reason, was known as "sleepwort" to the Anglo-Saxons. The dried juice of the lettuce was used as a sedative and hypnotic and also mixed with honey to treat a bad cough. Wild lettuce (*Lactuca virosa*) may retain these qualities in volume, while cultivated lettuce (*Lactuca sativa*) retains only a minor amount.

Natural Benefits
- aids normal elimination
- sedative
- helpful for:
  insomnia
  hair loss
  nervous problems

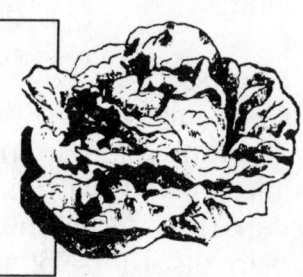

Cultivated lettuce has quantities of iron and magnesium, calcium, iodine, phosphorus, copper, cobalt, zinc, and potassium. Also vitamins A, C, D and E and the B-complex. Many of the therapeutic effects are attributed to the alkaloids present, which include asparagine, lactucine, lactucic acid, and own, hyoscyamine. Lettuce's silicon content helps promote the flexibility of muscles and joints.

Lemon

You may not have to use a juicer to get lemon juice, but the juice is too valuable not to be mentioned. It is one of the richest fruits in the bioflavonoid-vitamin C group. Lemon

skin cells, tissues, arteries and veins throughout the entire body. Capillary fragility, which causes gum bleeding and hard-to-heal wounds, can be traced to insufficient vitamin C and bioflavonoids

Lemons also contain potassium, calcium, phosphorus and iron as well as vitamin A and B-complex. The peels of lemons contain hesperidin, which helps the body absorb vitamin C. So when you do use your juicer, scrub the skin clean and juice it along with the pulp.

Mix lemon juice with water, half a lemon to a glass, otherwise the citric acid makes it umpalatable. Lemon juice every other day will help to keep you regular. Drink it before you have your breakfast.

> *Natural Benefits*
> - helpful for:
>   anemia
>   colds
>   constipation
>   cough
>   pyorrhea

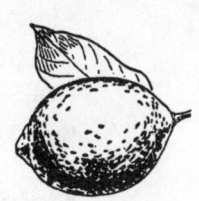

Lemon juice, undiluted, can be used to combat a sore throat. Take a tablespoonful and sip it.

Lime
Lemon's green cousin is very similar in nutrition and effect. It is less acidic than lemon but still a good body cleanser. Mix it with other juices for drinking unless you're using it

Mango

A multi-shaped tropical fruit related to cashew nuts, mango is luscious, juicy, orange-fleshed, with both rainbow-colored and yellow skin. It can be round, kidney-shaped, or long and narrow, ranging in size from a hen's egg to an ostrich's, weighing over five pounds. Green skin indicates that the fruit is not fully ripe, while black spots show that it is overripe. Ripe mangos will yield to pressure between your palms and almost-ripe ones will ripen in a couple of days in your home.

Mango skins can irritate your hands and your mouth. Peel the fruit by cutting it in half, removing the large seed inside, then strip off the skin. Mango juice is extremely high in vitamin A, C, magnesium, calcium and potassium.

If your store has loads of mangos, the not-so-ripe ones can be cooked or baked and eaten for their fiber content.

Melons

Melons come in all sizes, from the round muskmelon to the huge watermelon. They grow on sprawling vines with large, fuzzy leaves and are relatives of the squash and cucumber. The family includes cantaloupe, honeydew, casaba, Cranshaw, Persian, Santa Claus, and Spanish.

MELONS ARE RICH IN VITAMIN A AND C AND THE B-COMPLEX, WHICH MAKES THEM GOOD SKIN AND NERVE FOOD.

> *Natural Benefits*
> - tasty and stimulates the appetite
> - laxative
> - increase output of urine
> - rejuvenate tissue
> - helpful for:
>   skin problems
>   nerve problems

Melons are rich in vitamins A and C and the B-complex, which makes them good skin and nerve food.

Mushrooms

In Australia, some aboriginal people live almost entirely on mushrooms, which are commonly called "native bread." Healthful varieties are those which are firm, clean, moist and fresh. When exposed to light, mushrooms turn black, but if they are still firm, it will not diminish their nutrient content.

Mushrooms are rich in folic acid, pantothenic acid and phosphorus, as well as vitamins C and D. In addition, certain mushrooms such as the shiitake and reishi varieties are used for their ability to fight bacteria.

Mix mushroom juice with carrot and celery juice for best results.

Mustard

Mustard greens have a strong taste, but don't be put off by that because they have a load of nutritional sulphur for your skin. They also are loaded with vitamin C. So, mix them with spinach and carrot juice and you'll have a fantastic beverage for clear skin and extra capillary protection.

Nettles

The stinging nettle is usually thought of as a herb rather than as a vegetable to be juiced. However, the natural juice of nettles is very helpful when fragile capillaries result in bleeding from the gums. It is also valuable for the other end of the body—the juice, in small amounts, is useful to help heal hemorrhoids.

Natural Benefits
- diuretic for the kidneys
- helps eliminate uric acid
- helpful for:
  anemia
  bleeding of gums
  capillary fragility

The active elements are formic acid, gallic acid and histamine, plus a load of organic iron.

Orange

One glass of freshly squeezed orange juice can contain more than 750 units of vitamin A and 900 units of vitamin C. It is highly recommended by many nutritionists as an energy aid because of the natural sugar content. It also tones blood vessels and prevents brain fatigue. The brain runs on two sources of energy, sugar and glutamic acid. Without a constant supply, it can become hungry and fatigued, contributing to overall body fatigue, exhaustion and collapse.

Orange juice is also rich in calcium, iodine, phosphorus, potassium, sodium, chlorine and iron. Vitamins include A, C, and

> *Natural Benefits*
> - promotes normal digestion
> - combats infection
> - prevents scurvy
> - maintains the integrity of the blood vessels
> - rebuilds damaged skin and tissues
> - helps reduce fever
> - useful for:
>
> | | |
> |---|---|
> | colds | anemia |
> | gout | heart problems |
> | indigestion | weight loss |
> | rheumatism | pneumonia |
> | pyorrhea | |

the B-complex. Makes a delicious combination with grape, peach or nectarine juice.

Orange juice is a source of amino acids and provides trace elements such as silicon, zinc, manganese, chlorine and copper. It cleanses and tones the gastrointestinal tract and, although it is acidic in nature, it alkalizes the bloodstream.

Onion

One of our oldest known vegetables, the onion was an object of worship to the early Egyptians, and used by the Romans in treating skin disease and for healing wounds.

Many sanatoriums in Europe use onion juice as a tonic and digestive aid. Taken after a meal, the juice stimulates digestive action and the whole gastric tract.

Onions are rich in vitamin C, copper and iron, as well as sulphur, calcium and phosphorus. The darker the onion's skin the more pungent the taste of the juice. Unless it is being sipped to fight a throat infection, the juice is too strong to be taken on its own. Mix it in small amounts with other vegetable juice.

Papaya

A large pear-shaped fruit, papaya is sometimes called "the melon that grows on trees." Some papayas grow up to 18 inches long, but the most common length is about 6 inches. The smooth skin turns from yellow green to all yellow when it is ripe. The ripest papaya can have a skin of yellow-to-orange color and feel slightly soft to the touch.

Natural Benefits
- helpful for:

acidosis	acne
constipation	indigestion
ulcers	overweight
liver problems	kidney problems

Papaya flesh is similar to that of a muskmelon, but it sometimes has an almost peppery taste. In the center lie shiny, black peppercorn-size seeds which should be discarded.

An enzyme found in the skin and leaves is called papain. It is a proteolytic enzyme that makes digestion easier. Commercially, papain is extracted from the fruit and made into a powder for use as a digestant and as a meat tenderizer. If you are preparing the juice for an older person or for someone who is having trouble with their digestive system, buy and juice the unripe, green papaya because the unripe fruit contains more of the papain.

Papaya increases the body's blood coagulating ability, is a laxative, appetite stimulant and helps replace lost energy with its natural sugar content.

Parsley

Like garlic, cabbage, dandelions, carrots and leeks, parsley is one of our leading organic remedies. It's loaded with chlorophyll, vitamins A and C, and a host of minerals, including calcium, magnesium, phosphorus, potassium, sodium and sulphur.

> *Natural Benefits*
> - promotes normal digestion
> - eliminates uric acid
> - promotes urination
> - helpful for:
>   anemia
>   arthritis
>   bladder problems
>   female endocrine problems
>   kidney problems
>   liver problems
>   prostate problems
>   urinary tract problems

Parsley juice is useful as a body and blood cleanser. The juice is highly concentrated and must be mixed with other juices for palatability.

PARSLEY IS LOADED WITH CHLOROPHYLL, VITAMIN A AND C, AND A HOST OF MINERALS

Parsnip

This vegetable looks like a big white carrot. The two plants are related—both parsnips and carrots are members of the *Umbilliferae* family. The leaves of parsnip look like those of celery, another relative. Look for firm parsnips without double roots or knots. The small or medium-sized ones are the most flavorful, while the larger ones tend to have a woody taste and texture.

Natural Benefits
- helpful for:

acne	arthritis
asthma	bladder problems
cataracts	skin disorders

The juice is low in calcium but rich in potassium, phosphorus, sulphur, silicon and chlorine. Don't confuse the disinfectant chlorine used in pools and kitchen cleansers with the organic chlorine found in vegetables. This is a natural mineral that is used as a body cleanser. The combination of sulphur and silicon is very useful to the health of the skin and hair. A daily drink of parsnip juice mixed with carrot juice and a gentle buffing will restore damaged nails to their rightful healthy condition.

The juice is also particularly helpful to those suffering from lung conditions. The combination of chlorine and phosphorus does the job.

Passion Fruit
They are brownish-yellow or purple skinned, egg-shaped, with a strong flavor. They are full of small black seeds surrounded by golden orange flesh. Sounds good enough to eat!

> *Natural Benefits*
> - helps combat uric acid
> - mild laxative action
> - enhances normal intestinal functions
> - mild sedative
> - helpful for:
>   bladder problems   liver problems
>   prostate problems   urinary infections

Ripe passion fruit yields to gentle pressure and is loaded with nutritional values. The purple and sweet passion fruits are 3 to 6 inches in length and are more flavorful than the giant passion fruit.

Peach
The skin of the peach contains most of the nutritional value, so juice the whole peach after removing the pit. Peaches are exceptionally rich in vitamin A, With the average peach supplying 2000 units or more. They also contain good quantities of vitamin C and the B-complex as well as minerals such as

> *Natural Benefits*
> - provides energy
> - promotes normal stomach acidity
> - aids kidney function
> - has a gentle laxative action
> - can be used against "morning sickness"

calcium, potassium, manganese, chlorine, and sulphur.

The juice is an excellent cleanser for the lower bowel and is easy to digest.

Pear

Pears are cousins to the apple and have a similar seed core. The trees that bear pears have an exceptionally long life. They can bear fruit for 100 years or longer. The more popular varieties include Bartlett, Bosc, Anjou, Comice, and Winter Nelis (which are ripe when the skin is green with light brown spots.)

> TRY MIXING PEAR JUICE WITH APPLE JUICE, PLUS A BIT OF LEMON FOR A KICKER.

Pear juice may be a bit too thick for your liking, so try mixing it with apple juice, plus a bit of lemon for a kicker.

Pear juice contains vitamins A, B-complex, C, phosphorus, potassium, calcium, chlorine, iron, magnesium, sodium, and sulphur.

Peas

Pea juice is rich in protein and has a lot of vitamins A, C and B-complex. It also contains magnesium and phosphorus and is a good source of usable carbohydrate.

Drink the juice immediately after juicing, since the nutrient content is easily lost.

Peppers

Green peppers with firm, shiny skin, smooth and without wrinkles, are high in vitamins A and C. The greener the pepper, the higher the vitamin C content. The average pepper contains about 2500 units of vitamin A, high B-complex and. has less than 25 calories. The juice is rich in silicon, which nourishes your hair and nails. Skin blemishes, colic and annoying flatulence may be helped with pepper juice.

Persimmon

If you have your sunglasses on, you might think the persimmon was a tomato. However, its bright orange-red skin and flesh, with a green cap stem for a hat make the persimmon a very attractive fruit.

The "apple of the Orient" was born in Southeast Asia and, in a smaller form, in the southern United States. The Japanese call it *kaki*. It must be fully ripe before eating—that is, soft and slightly shriveled—since the tannic acid content in unripe fruit will make it very astringent and pucker up your mouth.

Pineapple

Noted for containing the digestant bromelain, which parallels the secretion of pancreatic hormones, the pineapple contains a protein-digesting enzyme to help assimilate food entering your digestive system. The thick skin contains a lot of nutrients, so be sure to squeeze out every last drop in your juicer.

PINEAPPLE CONTAINS A PROTEIN-DIGESTING ENZYME TO HELP ASSIMILATE FOOD.

The most nutritious pineapples are those which are a dark orange-yellow in color and heavy. The average pineapple contains loads of natural sugars for energy. Nutrients include vitamins A, B-complex and C, calcium, phosphorus, copper, iron and magnesium.

Natural Benefits
- easily digested nutrients
- regulates normal stomach acidity
- aids kidney function
- may enhance sexuality
- helpful for:
  colds
  gout
  pyorrhea
  sciatica
  overweight

The juice helps relieve the discomfort of a sore throat and bronchitis and helps to dissolve clumps of mucus. The citric and malic acids aid kidney function.

Plum
Plums, like their cousins peaches and cherries, are soft, roundish tree fruits with hard pits in the center. They have been eaten since the Stone Age.

Natural Benefits
- provides energy to muscles and nerves
- mild diuretic action
- aids normal elimination
- is a blood cleanser

Plums provide vitamin A, iron, potassium, calcium, and magnesium, as well as carbohydrates for energy. The *umeboshi* plums are used in Japan as a medicine. They are pickled in brine for two years, using a special antibacterial process. They are very salty and should not be eaten alone.

Pomegranate
This seedy "apple" is unique in that its hard, reddish-brown shell-skin contains a multitude of seeds, each surrounded by a juicy red pulp.

> *Natural Benefits*
> - heart stimulant
> - fights parasitic invasion
> - relieves diarrhea

Because the pulp and juice cling so hard to the seeds, juicing is the best way to get the most from your fruit.

Potato
The Spaniards discovered the potato growing in Peru about 1530 and brought it back to Europe, where it flourished in Spain and Italy. In France, potatoes were grown for use as an ornament until Parmentier in the eighteenth century popularized its use as a food. It wasn't easy because early potatoes had an acrid taste. Only through his work did potatoes become the tasty vegetable we enjoy. Because the stubborn Frenchmen still regarded the potato with suspicion, Parmentier resorted to

POTATOES CONTAIN VITAMIN A, B-COMPLEX, C, D, SODIUM, CALCIUM, MAGNESIUM, PHOSPHORUS, IRON, MANGANESE, COPPER AND SULPHUR.

> *Natural Benefits*
> - nutritious and easily digestible
> - good energy source
> - neutralizes stomach acid
> - aids healing
> - diuretic
> - helpful for:
>   arthritis
>   gastritis
>   peptic ulcers

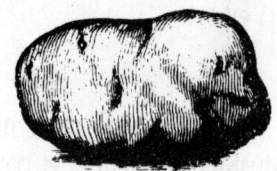

subterfuge. He planted potatoes in fields in the suburbs of Paris, then hired guards during the day to protect them. Naturally, the French invaded the fields during the unguarded night to pilfer the potatoes. It was not long before potatoes were being enjoyed throughout Paris and then all of France.

Potatoes contain vitamins A, B, C, D, sodium, calcium, magnesium, phosphorus, iron, manganese, copper, and sulphur.

Prunes

Prunes are dried plums, just as raisins are dried grapes. You can juice them, and you should because they will keep you regular. However, you need to use a a blender. Soak a handful of prunes in hot water overnight. Then, take the soaked prunes and the water and put them in the blender. Blend until pureed. You can take the juice as is or strain out the pulp for a clearer juice. The acids in prunes (quinic and benzoic acids) will give you a cleansing within a short period of time.

Prunes also contain good amounts of vitamin A, iron and copper

Prickly Pear

Not easy to find, but a valuable source of glucose and levulose as well as malic and tartaric acids.

> *Natural Benefit*
> - combats diarrhea

To avoid the constipating action of the seeds, use only the juice.

Quince

Contains vitamins A and B complex, cellulose, tannins and pectin.

Ratafia is a time-honored drink combining quince with other substances to combat indigestion, sour stomach and flatulence.

> *Natural Benefits*
> - combats diarrhea
> - stabilizes digestion
> - stimulates the appetite
> - aids liver function

Here's the recipe:

quince juice	1½ quarts
brandy	1 pint
cinnamon	2 grams
cloves	0.8 grams
bitter almonds	0.5 grams
mace	1 pinch

Soak for two months, filter and bottle.
Take a shot when necessary.

Radish

Nutritionists estimate the radish to be one-third potassium, one-third sodium and high in iron and magnesium. The juice helps stimulate your appetite, causes saliva to flow, and has an antiseptic effect on the intestinal tract. The high sulphur content tones the bloodstream and keeps it fresh and clean. It heals and soothes the mucous membranes. Because the juice is very strong, it should be mixed with other juices. Carrot juice and radish juice make a great combination.

Natural Benefits
- promotes gall bladder function
- stimulates respiration
- enhances appetite and digestion
- aids diuresis
- calms the nerves
- helpful for:
  asthma   eczema
  lung problems   sinus problems
  thyroid disorders (contains iodine)

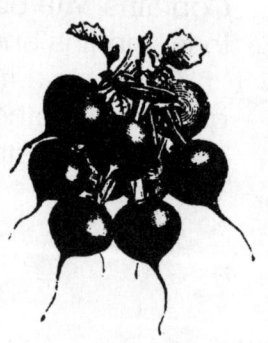

Radish juice also contains vitamin C. If you can get radish sprouts, you can juice them as well. Take a handful and run it through the juicer along with other greens or with carrot juice. Radish sulphur helps clear up skin blemishes.

Scallion

Like the other pungent-flavored juices, that of the green onion is highly cleansing for the mucous membranes of the lungs and digestive and respiratory tracts. It is also a stimulant to the circulatory system, heart and digestion.

> *Natural Benefits*
> - promotes weight loss
> - helpful for:
>   asthma   coughs
>   infection   stuffed nose
>   skin problems   nervous problems

Small amounts of the juice mixed with other green vegetable juices can be a welcome beginning to a meal. It gets your juices flowing and is warming to the stomach.

Spinach

Spinach is exceptionally high in vitamins A and C. Its iron content is in a form that is readily useful to your body. However, spinach also contains oxalic acid, which may interfere with calcium absorption.

It's a great body cleanser and tissue builder with an ample supply of chlorophyll, magnesium, phosphorus, potassium, sodium, and trace elements. It is mildly laxative in nature, particularly when mixed with other green juices.

Teeth and gums love spinach because it contains a high concentration of alkaline minerals.

> *Natural Benefits*
> - combats anemia
> - aids normal heart function
> - helpful for:
>   circulatory weakness colitis
>   eye problems   kidney problems
>   liver problems   nervous problems
>   pyorrhea   poor digestion
>   skin problems   thyroid problems

Strawberry

By far the most popular berry in the United States is the strawberry. How it got its name is unknown. Maybe because they used straw as a mulch around the strawberry plants.

Natural Benefits
- laxative
- promotes urine production
- enhances the elimination of uric acid
- helps lower blood pressure
- promotes normal metabolism of the liver, endocrine glands, and nervous system
- helpful for:
  kidney problems
  rheumatism
  thyroid problems

They should be fully red, slightly soft and fragrant, with stems intact. To retain the sweet juice, do not remove the green caps until you have washed them. Drain the strawberries stem side down on absorbent paper. Store uncovered in the refrigerator.

Strawberries contain vitamins A, C, B-complex, E and K, plus iron, sodium, phosphorus, magnesium, potassium, sulphur, calcium, silicon, iodine and bromine.

Tangerine

The tangerine is related to the orange, but is not as rich in minerals. Its distinctive virtue is sedation due to the high bromine content. When juicing, try to include the inner portion of the skin, since the vitamin C and bioflavonoids are concentrated there.

Tomato

The tomato is a predominantly alkaline vegetable (fruit), due to its mineral content. It helps to neutralize excessively acid stomach conditions caused by the ingestion of too much starch. The piquant flavor and delicious-appearing red color adds zest to any meal. It is one of the best sources of vitamins C and B2, as well as a load of vegetable amino acids iron, potassium, magnesium and phosphorus.

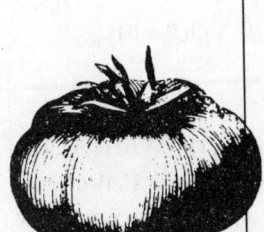

Natural Benefits
- provides energy
- enhances cellular metabolism
- stimulates appetite
- aids diuresis
- enhances normal bowel activity
- aids digestion
- helpful for:
  bladder problems   skin problems
  gout   liver problems
  gall bladder problems

Maybe it's neither a fruit nor a vegetable...maybe it's a berry!

In 1893, the Supreme Court of the United States officially designated it as a vegetable because fruits were allowed to be imported without duty. So it was a question of money.

Turnips

Don't throw out the greens. Juice them for their high calcium content. Ounce for ounce, turnip greens contain more calcium than milk!

The root is no slouch either. It has calcium, potassium, phosphorus, magnesium, sulphur, iodine, copper, vitamins A, B-com-

> **Natural Benefits**
> - provides energy
> - aids diuresis
> - eliminates uric acid
> - helpful for:
>   anemia   arthritis
>   bladder problems   bronchitis
>   circulatory problems eye problems
>   infections   kidney problems
>   skin problems   lung problems

plex and C. Put them together in the juicer and you have a nutritional cocktail.

Build stronger bones, hair, nails and teeth. Mix the juice with alfalfa sprouts, dandelion greens, parsley, cabbage, spinach and sweet pepper...drink and jump-start your day.

Watercress

Watercress grows beside streams with sandy beds. It is a wild herb with a tangy flavor. Its rich green leaves are abundant with minerals. One-third of watercress is pure sulphur. The juice is acid-forming and should be mixed with carrot or celery juice. It acts as an intestinal cleanser and aid in the normal process of blood regeneration.

> **Natural Benefits**
> - helpful for:
>   anemia
>   bladder problems
>   circulatory problems
>   intestinal problems
>   kidney problems
>   liver problems
>   skin problems
>   endocrine imbalance (female)

The vitamin content includes A, B-complex and C. Chlorophyll lovers will take to this juice with glee. Minerals in watercress include calcium, potassium and phosphorus. Its high sulphur content assures proper pancreas gland function and the readily available manganese is a stimulant to the pituitary gland. Stimulating to the digestive system, it is useful to those who have difficulty digesting their food.

Watermelon

When you juice a watermelon you use everything, pulp, rind and seeds, so be sure you wash the fruit well.

Watermelon juice is loaded with vitamin A and potassium as well as substantial amounts of other vitamins, minerals and chlorophyll. The juice is excellent for flushing out the kidneys and bladder. It can be helpful during menstruation, when excess water can be uncomfortable.

When it's in season, you can use the juice several times a day, since it restores liquid to the body and then helps it run through, taking out waste material.

Like all raw fruits and vegetables, it is loaded with natural enzymes and is easy to digest.

Natural Benefits
- helpful for:
  arthritis   bladder problems
  constipation   fluid retention
  kidney problems   prostate problems
  skin problems

FRUIT PREPARATION FOR BEST NUTRITIOUS JUICING

If you can't find organic fruit, try to get an all-natural biodegradable cleanser and wash the produce thoroughly to remove surface sprays and pesticides.

❧ Apples
Rub or scrub your apple until clean. If you have to buy waxed fruit, remove the skin before juicing. If you are lucky enough to have organic apples, you can use all of the fruit. Core the apple to remove the seeds. Slice into juicing size pieces and juice.

❧ Apricots
Clean the fruit and remove the stem and the pit. When apricots are juiced, they produce a thick juice called a nectar. To make a thinner juice for drinking, mix the apricot juice with apple juice.

It's tough to juice a banana.

❧ Bananas
It's tough to juice a banana. If you try you'll only end up with mush. Instead, use a ripe banana in your blender and add apple or any other fruit juice. Banana is one of the few fruits which contain chromium.

❧ Blackberries
Wash berries thoroughly before juicing. An easy way to wash them is in a sieve or strainer.

❧ Blueberries
Wash well and serve freshly juiced to preserve the nutritional contents. Here's another fruit with chromium.

❧ Cantaloupe
If you scrub the skin very well and are sure it's clean, you can use everything in the juicer. Just cut into strips and feed the juicer, then feed your face.

❧ Cherries
Wash the cherries well, remove the pits and juice.

❧ Cranberries
Wash and juice.

❧ Grapefruit
The white underskin contains important factors and should be included in your juice procedure. Carefully pare the outer skin away, leaving the white intact. Cut in sections and juice.

❧ Grapes
Don't bother to remove the grapes from the stem. Just wash them well and juice the whole bunch.

❧ Lemon or lime
Don't peel them. Clean the skins, cut into small wedges and juice.

❧ Oranges
As with grapefruit, the white underpeel is important. Pare the outer skin, cut into sections and juice. One more fruit which contains chromium.

❧ Peaches
Wash, remove pit and juice.

❧ Pears
Scrub the skin well and core. Cut into juicing size and juice.

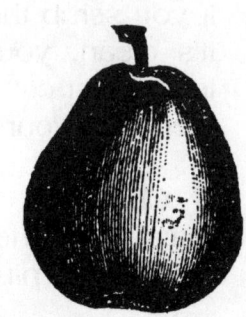

❧ Plums
Wash well, remove pit and juice.

❧ Pomegranate
Scrub the outer skin until clean then cut into small wedges, seeds and all, and juice.

❧ Raspberries
Wash well and juice.

❧ Strawberries
Wash well, remove green tops and juice. Once again, chromium.

❧ Tangerines
Peel as carefully as you can to try to save the underpeel, then juice.

❧ Watermelon
Wash the skin very well, then use everything, rind, pulp, seeds in your juicer.

VEGETABLE PREPARATION FOR BEST NUTRITIONAL JUICING

🌿 Alfalfa or bean sprouts
Rinse fresh sprouts in water and pat dry. Take any leafy green vegetable and roll sprouts in it for best and most complete juicing.

🌿 Asparagus
Clean the spears with a soft brush and trim off 1 inch from the bottom to get rid of dirt. Juice the entire spear or steam the soft part and juice the stalk.

🌿 Beans, string
Just wash and juice, don't trim.

🌿 Beets
Scrub with a firm brush and cut into suitable size for juicing.

🌿 Beet greens
Wash and juice with or without beet root.

🌿 Broccoli
Wash and shake dry. Cut into juicing size and juice.

🌿 Brussels sprouts
Remove old leaves and bad spots. Cut to juicing size after thorough washing.

🌿 Cabbage
Remove old or damaged leaves, rinse under running water and cut to juicing size.

❧ Carrots
Scrub clean and remove both ends. Cut to size and juice.

❧ Cauliflower
Clean and trim. Remove any dark or dry areas. Cut to juicing size.

❧ Celery
Clean and remove any bad areas. Leaves can be juiced with stalks, but they tend to be bitter.

❧ Chard, Swiss
Wash and shake dry. Wrap leaves around other vegetables you're using for juicing.

❧ Cucumbers
If waxed, remove the skin. Wash before juicing. If cucumbers tend to make you gassy, split down the middle and remove the seeds before juicing.

❧ Dandelion greens
Rinse in cold water to remove dirt. Cut or tear to juicing size.

❧ Garlic
Peel clove and juice.

❧ Ginger
Cut thin slices and add to juicer.

ॐ Kale
Rinse in cold water and juice.

ॐ Leeks
Rinse and trim off dirty end. Cut to size.

ॐ Onions
Remove outer skin and cut into wedges for juicing.

ॐ Parsley
Rinse and shake dry. Wrap in the leaf of another vegetable. Use plunger to push down into juicer.

ॐ Peppers, Bell/sweet
Clean and slice but don't bother to remove the seeds. Slice and juice.

ॐ Potatoes
Scrub clean, remove any dark spots or eyes. Slice into juicing size and juice.

ॐ Radishes
Scrub clean and juice.

ॐ Spinach
Rinse and shake dry. Wrap around other veggies for juicing.

ॐ Turnips
Scrub clean and cut to size for juicing.

ॐ Watercress
Rinse and gently shake dry. Wrap with other vegetables and push into juicer.

AVAILABILITY AND STORAGE OF FRESH FRUITS

Storage temperature:
Refrigerate unless otherwise noted

Fruit	Availability	Peak	Maximum Storage Time
Apples	year-round	Sept.–Nov.	1 week or more at 32°–34° F
Apricots	June–Sept.	June–July	3 to 5 days
Avocados	year-round	Oct.–Jan.	3 to 5 days at 65°–70° (unripe)
Bananas	year-round		1 to 5 days at room temp.
Blackberries	July–Sept.	July–Aug.	1 or 2 days
Blueberries	June–Aug.	July–Aug.	3 to 5 days
Cherries	June–Aug.	June	1 or 2 days
Cranberries	Sept.–Dec.	November	1 week
Currants	June–Aug.	July	1 or 2 days
Dates	year-round	November	
Figs, fresh	July–Oct.	July–Oct.	1 or 2 days
Gooseberries	May–Aug.	June–July	1 or 2 days
Grapefruits	year-round	Jan.–Apr.	1 week
Grapes	June–Mar.	summer	3 to 5 days
Kiwi fruit	year-round	June–Mar.	4 to 6 months
Kumquats	May–Aug.	Nov.–Feb.	5 days
Lemons	year-round	May–Aug.	5 days
Limes	year-round	June–Sept.	5 days
Mandarins	Nov.–May	Nov.–Jan.	5 days

Fruit	Availability	Peak	Maximum Storage Time
Mangos	Jan.–Aug.	June	3–5 days at room temp.
Melons			
Honeydew	June–Dec.	July–Oct.	3 to 5 days
Muskmelon	May–Nov.	July–Oct.	3 to 5 days
Watermelon	May–Oct.	June–Aug.	3 to 5 days
Nectarines	May–Sept.	July–Aug.	3 to 5 days
Oranges	year-round	Dec.–Mar.	5 days
Papayas	May–June; Oct.–Dec.	May, Oct.	1 week
Peaches	May–Sept.	July–Aug.	3 to 5 days
Pears	July–Mar.	July–Mar.	3 to 5 days
Persimmons	Apr.–June	Sept.–Jan.	3 to 5 days
Pineapples	year-round	Apr.–June	1 to 2 days
Plums	May–Sept.	July–Aug.	3 to 5 days
Pomegranates	Aug.–Dec.	October	1 week
Raspberries	June–Sept.	July–Aug.	1 or 2 days
Rhubarb	Apr.–June	Apr.–June	2–3 weeks
Strawberries	year-round	Nov.–Jan.	1 or 2 days
Tangelos	Oct.–Apr.	Nov.–Jan.	5 days
Tangerines	Oct.–Mar.		5 days

AVAILABILITY AND STORAGE OF FRESH VEGETABLES

Name	Availability	Peak	Imported From	Storage Temp
Artichokes, globe	all year	Mar.–May		32–35°
Artichokes, Jerusalem	Oct.–Mar.			32–35°
Asparagus	Feb.–July	Apr.–June	Mexico	32–35°
Beans	all year	May–Aug.		45–50°
Beets	all year	June–Oct.		32–35° (cut off tops)
Broccoli	all year	Oct.–May		32–35°
Brussels sprouts	all year	Oct.–Mar.		32–35°
Cabbage	all year			32–35"
Carrots	all year		Canada	32–35° (cut off tops)
Cauliflower	all year	Sept.–Jan.		32–35° (stem side up)
Celery	all year			32–35°
Collards	all year			32–35°
Corn, sweet	all year	May–Aug.		32°
Cucumbers	all year	May–July	Mexico	45–50°
Eggplant	all year	Aug.–Sept.	Mexico	45–50°
Garlic	all year		Italy, Spain	32° (in a dry area)
Kale	all year	Dec.–Feb.		32–35°

Name	Availability	Peak	Imported From	Storage Temp
Leeks	all year	Oct.–June		32–35°
Lettuce	all year			32–35°
Mushrooms	all year			33–40°
Mustard greens	all year	Dec.–Apr.		32–35°
Okra	June–Nov.	July		40–50°
Onions, dry	all year			65–70° (in a dry area)
Onions, green	all year			32–35°
Parsley	all year			32–35°
Parsnips	all year	Jan.–Apr.		32–35°
Peas	Mar.–Sept.	Mar.–June		32–35°
Peppers	all year	June–July	Mexico	45–50°
Potatoes	all year		Canada	45–55° (dark, dry area)
Radishes	all year	Mar.–May		32–35°
Rutabagas	all year	Oct.–Feb.		60°
Spinach	all year	Dec.–May		32–35°
Squash, summer	all year	May–July		45–50°
Squash, winter	Aug.–Mar.	Oct.–Dec.		50–55°
Sweet potatoes (yams)	all year	Sept.–Jan.		55–60°
Tomatoes	all year	May–July	Mexico	50–70°
Turnips	all year	Oct.–Mar.		32–35°
Watercress	all year	May–Oct.		32–35°

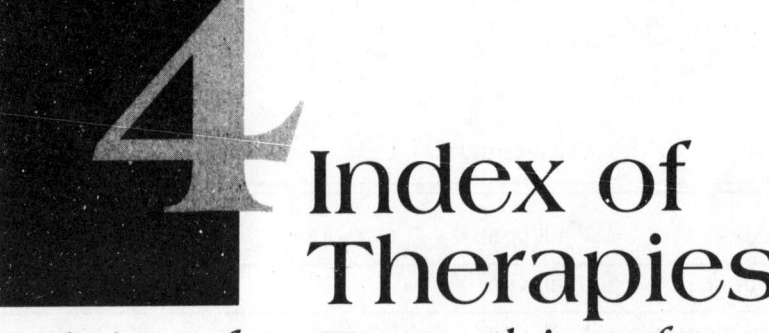

4 Index of Therapies
Juicing for Everything from Acne to Water Retention

The following formulas are listed here as a guide for the healing profession and as general information. They are based on folkloric reports and centuries of usage, and even though modern research is proving the value of juice combinations, these are not intended to be prescriptive. Juice therapy may be adjunctive with prescriptions written by your health professional.

✿ Acne

1.	Carrot juice	16 ounces
2	Carrot juice	6 ounces
	spinach juice	6 ounces
	lettuce juice	4 ounces

Drink daily in divided doses.

3. Carrot juice   10 ounces
   spinach juice   6 ounces
Drink daily in divided doses.

4. Asparagus juice   6 ounces
Drink daily when acne is accompanied by water retention.

NOTE: Several juice mixtures are given for some conditions. It is not necessary to use all the combinations. Try one combination for a week and observe the results, then try another. Use up to 16 ounces daily of the combination which proves best suited to your individual body chemistry.

❧ Acidosis

1. Carrot juice   10 ounces
   spinach juice   6 ounces

2. Carrot juice   10 ounces
   beet juice   3 ounces
   cucumber juice   3 ounces

❧ Addison's Disease

1. Carrot juice   7 ounces
   lettuce juice   5 ounces
   pomegranate juice   4 ounces

2. Celery juice   7 ounces
   lettuce juice   5 ounces
   spinach juice   4 ounces

Adenoids

In this condition a combination of juices is suggested:

1. Carrot juice	16 ounces

Daily plus one of the following mixtures:

2. Comfrey juice	10 ounces
horseradish (grated)	1 ounce

3. Onion juice	6 ounces
garlic juice	1/2 ounce
horseradish (grated)	1 ounce

Sip at intervals throughout the day.

4. Spinach juice	8 ounces
dandelion juice	4 ounces
comfrey juice	4 ounces

Allergy

1. Carrot juice	10 ounces
spinach juice	6 ounces

2. Carrot juice	8 ounces
beet root juice	8 ounces

3. Carrot juice	8 ounces
tomato juice	8 ounces

4. Carrot juice	12 ounces
celery juice	4 ounces

Albuminuria

1. Carrot juice	11 ounces
beet juice	3 ounces
coconut milk	2 ounces

2.	Carrot juice	9 ounces
	celery juice	5 ounces
	parsley juice	2 ounces

| 3. | Carrot juice | 12 ounces |
| | parsley juice | 4 ounces |

Anemia

(Simple anemia, not pernicious anemia, which requires the assistance of an M.D.)

| 1. | Carrot juice | 9 ounces |
| | fennel juice | 7 ounces |

2.	Carrot juice	10 ounces
	dandelion juice	3 ounces
	turnip juice	3 ounces

3.	Carrot juice	6 ounces
	fennel juice	6 ounces
	beetroot juice	4 ounces

4.	Watercress juice	2 ounces
	spinach juice	13 ounces
	horseradish (grated)	1 ounce

Angina

1.	Carrot juice	7 ounces
	celery juice	4 ounces
	parsley juice	2 ounces
	spinach juice	3 ounces

2.	Carrot juice	10 ounces
	beet juice	3 ounces
	cucumber juice	3 ounces

Apoplexy

1.	Carrot juice	10 ounces
	spinach juice	6 ounces

2.	Carrot juice	8 ounces
	spinach juice	4 ounces
	turnip juice	2 ounces
	watercress juice	2 ounces

Antibiotic Therapy

RESTORE THE GASTRIC FLORA WITH YOGURT AND JUICE MIXTURES.

Because helpful bacteria as well as harmful ones are destroyed during antibiotic therapy, you must be careful to restore the gastric flora. Eat yogurt daily and drink 6 ounces of any of the following mixtures in divided doses throughout the day for three days:

1.	Apple juice	16 ounces

2.	Papaya juice	16 ounces

3.	Cucumber juice	10 ounces
	garlic juice	1/2 ounce
	onion juice	1/2 ounce
	carrot juice	5 ounces

Artery Health

Walk a lot, take a complete vitamin supplement with extra vitamin E. Start with formula 1 and take a different mixture daily.

1.	Carrot juice	10 ounces
	spinach juice	6 ounces

2.	Carrot juice	8 ounces
	beetroot juice	4 ounces
	celery juice	4 ounces

3.	Carrot juice	8 ounces
	celery juice	4 ounces
	spinach juice	2 ounces
	parsley juice	2 ounces
4.	Carrot juice	8 ounces
	nettle juice	8 ounces
5.	Pineapple juice	6 ounces
	garlic juice	2 ounces
	carrot juice	8 ounces
6.	Pineapple juice	8 ounces
	papaya juice	8 ounces
7.	Horseradish	1 ounce
	garlic juice	2 ounces
	carrot juice	13 ounces
8.	Carrot juice	8 ounces
	lettuce juice	4 ounces
	spinach juice	4 ounces

Arthritis

Take up to two pints of celery juice daily plus one of the following combinations:

1.	Spinach juice	8 ounces
	parsley juice	2 ounces
	cucumber juice	6 ounces
2.	Spinach juice	8 ounces
	parsley juice	2 ounces
	nettle juice	6 ounces
3.	Grapefruit juice	16 ounces
4.	Carrot juice	10 ounces
	spinach juice	6 ounces

5.	Carrot juice	10 ounces
	beet juice	3 ounces
	cucumber juice	3 ounces

Asthma

Try a number of different combinations to see which one benefits you most.

1.	Spinach juice	8 ounces
	parsley juice	2 ounces
	cucumber juice	6 ounces
2.	Spinach juice	8 ounces
	parsley juice	2 ounces
	nettle juice	6 ounces
3.	Grapefruit juice	16 ounces
4.	Carrot juice	10 ounces
	spinach juice	6 ounces

Backache

1.	Carrot juice	10 ounces
	beet juice	3 ounces
	cucumber juice	3 ounces
2.	Carrot juice	10 ounces
	spinach juice	6 ounces
3.	Carrot juice	10 ounces
	cranberry juice	6 ounces

Bedwetting

1.	Carrot juice	10 ounces
	beet juice	3 ounces
	cucumber juice	3 ounces

2. Carrot juice — 10 ounces
   beet juice — 3 ounces
   coconut milk — 3 ounces
   To be taken at intervals during the day but not later than 6 p.m.

Biliousness

The failure of the body to produce enough bile to digest all the fat in the diet. Avoid fried foods, excess fats and alcoholic beverages.

1. Carrot juice — 10 ounces
   celery juice — 4 ounces
   parsley juice — 2 ounces

2. Cucumber juice — 4 ounces
   carrot juice — 8 ounces
   beetroot juice — 4 ounces

3. Dandelion juice — 8 ounces
   watercress juice — 2 ounces
   nettle juice — 4 ounces

4. Carrot juice — 10 ounces
   spinach juice — 6 ounces

Bladder Trouble

1. Carrot juice — 10 ounces
   beet juice — 3 ounces
   cucumber juice — 3 ounces

2. Carrot juice — 10 ounces
   spinach juice — 6 ounces

3. Cranberry juice — 16 ounces

4. Blueberry juice — 8 ounces
   cranberry juice — 8 ounces

Blood Pressure (high)

1.	Carrot juice	7 ounces
	celery juice	4 ounces
	parsley juice	2 ounces
	spinach juice	3 ounces
2.	Carrot juice	10 ounces
	beet juice	3 ounces
	cucumber juice	3 ounces

Blood Pressure (low)

1.	Carrot juice	10 ounces
	beet juice	3 ounces
	coconut milk	2 ounces
2.	Carrot juice	10 ounces
	beet juice	3 ounces
	cucumber juice	3 ounces

Boils

1.	Carrot juice	8 ounces
	lettuce juice	5 ounces
	spinach juice	3 ounces

Bone and Teeth Health

Take a pint a day of any combination of these:

1. Beetroot leaves juice
2. Cabbage juice
3. Celery juice
4. Chard juice
5. Dandelion leaves juice

6. Kale juice

7. Leek juice

8. Parsley juice (no more than 4 ounces mixed with other juices)

9. Turnip greens juice

10. Watercress juice (no more than ounces mixed with other juices)

Bronchitis

1. Horseradish, grated — 2 ounces
   lemon juice — 2 ounces
   water — 12 ounces

2. Turnip juice — 10 ounces
   lemon juice — 4 ounces
   water — 2 ounces

3. Cabbage juice — 14 ounces
   garlic juice — 2 ounces

4. To help cut mucus:
   pineapple juice — 8 ounces
   Gargle, then swallow a bit at a time.

5. To help restore strength:
   carrot juice — 10 ounces
   beetroot juice — 5 ounces
   cucumber juice — 1 ounce

Bursitis

1. Carrot juice — 8 ounces
   radish juice — 4 ounces
   watercress juice — 4 ounces

2.	Carrot juice	10 ounces
	spinach juice	6 ounces

Chronic Catarrh

1.	Horseradish, grated	4 ounces
	lemon juice	2 ounces
	water	12 ounces
2.	Papaya juice	8 ounces
	pineapple juice	4 ounces
	grapefruit juice	4 ounces
3.	Carrot juice	10 ounces
	radish juice	4 ounces
	parsley juice	2 ounces

Chicken Pox

1.	Carrot juice	10 ounces
	beet juice	3 ounces
	cucumber juice	3 ounces
2.	Carrot juice	7 ounces
	celery juice	4 ounces
	parsley juice	2 ounces
	spinach juice	3 ounces

Chorea

Carrot juice	9 ounces
celery juice	3 ounces
parsley juice	2 ounces

Cirrhosis

1.	Carrot juice	10 ounces
	beet juice	3 ounces
	cucumber juice	3 ounces
2.	Carrot juice	10 ounces
	spinach juice	6 ounces

Circulation

1.	Horseradish, grated	3 ounces
	carrot juice	13 ounces
2.	Carrot juice	14 ounces
	garlic juice	1 ounce
	onion juice	1 ounce
3.	Pineapple juice	10 ounces
	grapefruit juice	3 ounces
	papaya juice	3 ounces

Colds

1.	Carrot juice	12 ounces
	radish juice	4 ounces
2.	Carrot juice	7 ounces
	celery juice	6 ounces
	radish juice	3 ounces
3.	Carrot juice	9 ounces
	beet juice	3 ounces
	cucumber juice	4 ounces
4.	Carrot juice	10 ounces
	spinach juice	6 ounces
5.	orange juice	16 ounces

6. Pineapple juice	10 ounces
grapefruit juice	6 ounces

Colic

1. Carrot juice	10 ounces
spinach juice	6 ounces
2. Carrot juice	10 ounces
beet juice	3 ounces
cucumber juice	3 ounces

Colitis

Increase your intake of bran and explore these juice combinations:

1. Apple juice	10 ounces
carrot juice	6 ounces
2. Beet juice	8 ounces
carrot juice	4 ounces
cucumber juice	4 ounces
3. Papaya juice	16 ounces
4. Carrot juice	10 ounces
spinach juice	6 ounces

Constipation

1. Prune juice	6 ounces
lemon juice	3 ounces
carrot juice	7 ounces
2. Carrot juice	8 ounces
apple juice	8 ounces
3. Potato juice	16 ounces

4.	Carrot juice	9 ounces
	beet juice	4 ounces
	cucumber juice	3 ounces

Cramps (intestinal)

1.	Carrot juice	10 ounces
	beet juice	3 ounces
	cucumber juice	3 ounces

Cystitis

1.	Cranberry juice	8 ounces
	blueberry juice	8 ounces
2.	Carrot juice	9 ounces
	celery juice	5 ounces
	parsley	2 ounces
3.	Carrot juice	12 ounces
	green pepper juice	4 ounces

Convalescence

All juices are helpful, since they are easy to digest. Drink as much as you can and still be comfortable.

Dermatitis

1.	Carrot juice	6 ounces
	apple juice	6 ounces
	celery juice	4 ounces
2.	Carrot juice	8 ounces
	celery juice	8 ounces

3.	Carrot juice	10 ounces
	parsley juice	2 ounces
	watercress juice	4 ounces

Diabetes
Helpful juices include:

| 1. | Brussels sprout juice | 8 ounces |
| | string bean juice | 8 ounces |

2.	Carrot juice	6 ounces
	lettuce juice	4 ounces
	string bean juice	3 ounces
	Brussels sprout juice	3 ounces

3.	Lemon juice	2 ounces
	horseradish (grated)	2 ounces
	water	12 ounces

4.	Carrot juice	9 ounces
	celery juice	5 ounces
	parsley juice	2 ounces

Diarrhea

1.	Carrot juice	7 ounces
	celery juice	4 ounces
	parsley juice	2 ounces
	spinach juice	3 ounces

| 2. | Cabbage juice | 8 ounces |
| | beet juice | 8 ounces |

3.	Cabbage juice	6 ounces
	garlic juice	1 ounce
	nettle juice	7 ounces

4.	Papaya juice	8 ounces
	pineapple juice	8 ounces
5.	Blackberry juice	8 ounces
	carrot juice	8 ounces

Dysentery
Use any of the above formulas, but drink at least 4 pints a day to replace lost water.

Dyspepsia (see Indigestion)

Dysuria
Painful or difficult urination.

Blueberry juice	8 ounces
cranberry juice	8 ounces

Eczema
Not so much a disease as a symptom. Often brought on by stress, sometimes due to diet or alcohol.

1.	Spinach juice	5 ounces
	carrot juice	11 ounces
2.	Potato juice	10 ounces
3.	Carrot juice	7 ounces
	celery juice	4 ounces
	parsley juice	2 ounces
	spinach juice	3 ounces
4.	Carrot juice	9 ounces
	beet juice	3 ounces
	lettuce juice	4 ounces

5.	Papaya juice	12 ounces
6.	Nettle juice	4 ounces
	carrot juice	10 ounces
	lettuce juice	2 ounces

Emphysema

Watercress juice	2 ounces
potato juice	4 ounces
carrot juice	7 ounces
parsnip juice	3 ounces

Erysipelas

Carrot juice	9 ounces
celery juice	5 ounces
parsley juice	2 ounces

Eye Problems

All eye problems should be brought to the attention of your physician. Those problems brought about by nutrient deficiency and/or free radical attack may respond to juice therapy.

1.	Carrot juice	10 ounces
	fennel juice	6 ounces
2.	Carrot juice	12 ounces
	parsley juice	1 ounce
	watercress juice	3 ounces
3.	Carrot juice	8 ounces
	celery juice	8 ounces

4.	Papaya juice	12 ounces
	grapefruit juice	4 ounces
5.	Carrot juice	8 ounces
	spinach juice	2 ounces
	melon juice	6 ounces

Fatigue

If it is chronic, fatigue may be an indication that your body is not getting the energy it needs from your diet. It can also be the precursor of a disease, or the result of stress and anxiety. Raw juices can supply nascent power but if your condition does not respond, see a health professional.

1.	Grapefruit juice in divided doses	16 ounces
2.	Orange juice in divided doses	16 ounces
3.	Grapefruit juice	8 ounces
	lemon juice	2 ounces
	orange juice	6 ounces
4.	Carrot juice	10 ounces
	spinach juice	6 ounces
5.	Carrot juice	10 ounces
	beet juice	3 ounces
	cucumber juice	3 ounces
6.	Orange juice	8 ounces
	apple juice	6 ounces
	lettuce juice	1 ounce
	lemon juice	1 ounce

Fever

Fever is the body's effort to burn out unwanted visiting organisms. Carefully controlled fever can shorten colds or the flu. Try it with your doctor's supervision.

Drink all the raw fruit juice you can get down, and try this formula:

Cabbage juice	10 ounces
carrot juice	4 ounces

Also, drink all you can of citrus fruit juices, grape juice, or mixtures of vegetable and fruit juices.

Fractures

Raw juice mixtures can supply the calcium and other nutrients the body uses to heal broken bones.

1.	Carrot juice	8 ounces
	whole milk	8 ounces
2.	Carrot juice	8 ounces
	comfrey juice	8 ounces

Gall bladder problems

These require your doctor's advice. Meanwhile, avoid fatty or fried foods and lose some weight.

1.	Apple juice	10 ounces
	celery juice	6 ounces
2.	Carrot juice	10 ounces
	beet juice	3 ounces
	coconut milk	3 ounces

3.	Carrot juice	10 ounces
	cumber juice	3 ounces
	beet juice	3 ounces
4.	Carrot juice	10 ounces
	spinach juice	6 ounces
5.	Carrot juice	8 ounces
	nettle juice	4 ounces
	watercress juice	4 ounces

Gastritis

1.	Carrot juice	10 ounces
	spinach juice	6 ounces
2.	Carrot juice	10 ounces
	apple juice	3 ounces
	cucumber juice	3 ounces

Goiter

Needs treatment by a physician, since a lack of iodine may be the cause. Your doctor may add kelp, dulse or other forms of organic iodine to your diet.

1.	Parsley juice	1 ounce
	carrot juice	8 ounces
	celery juice	7 ounces
2.	Carrot juice	8 ounces
	celery juice	4 ounces
	spinach juice	4 ounces
3	Carrot juice	10 ounces
	spinach juice	6 ounces

4.	Watercress juice	2 ounces
	spinach juice	4 ounces
	carrot juice	10 ounces

Gout

Your doctor may advise no wine or beer, no anchovies, no sardines, very little meat. Try a vegetarian diet for a month to see how you feel.

1.	String bean juice	6 ounces
2.	Carrot juice	10 ounces
	celery juice	4 ounces
	parsley juice	2 ounces
3.	Cherry juice	4 ounces
	carrot juice	12 ounces
4.	Spinach juice	6 ounces
	carrot juice	6 ounces
	celery juice	4 ounces

Hair health

1.	Alfalfa sprout juice	6 ounces
	lettuce juice	4 ounces
	carrot juice	6 ounces
2.	Spinach juice	8 ounces
	carrot juice	8 ounces

Hay fever

1.	Celery juice	8 ounces
	carrot juice	8 ounces

2.	Beet juice	6 ounces
	cucumber juice	4 ounces
	carrot juice	6 ounces
3.	Horseradish (grated)	2 ounces
	lemon juice	1 ounce
	water	12 ounces
4.	Carrot juice	6 ounces
	celery juice	6 ounces
	spinach juice	2 ounces
	parsley juice	2 ounces

Headache

1.	Apple juice	8 ounces
	parsley juice	2 ounces
	tomato juice	6 ounces
2.	Cabbage juice	12 ounces
	celery juice	4 ounces
3.	Carrot juice	8 ounces
	beet juice	4 ounces
	cucumber juice	4 ounces
4.	Cabbage juice	10 ounces
	beet juice	6 ounces

Hemorrhoids

1.	Potato juice	8 ounces
	watercress juice	4 ounces
	carrot juice	4 ounces
2.	Carrot juice	10 ounces
	spinach juice	6 ounces

3.	Turnip juice	2 ounces
	watercress juice	2 ounces
	carrot juice	12 ounces
4.	Nettle juice	1 ounce

Take after meals and at bedtime.

Indigestion

1.	Cabbage juice	10 ounces
	celery juice	6 ounces
2.	Papaya juice	16 ounces
3.	Carrot juice	10 ounces
	beet juice	3 ounces
	cucumber juice	3 ounces
4.	Carrot juice	10 ounces
	spinach juice	6 ounces
5.	Pineapple juice	16 ounces
6.	Tomato juice	16 ounces
7	Carrot juice	7 ounces
	beet juice	6 ounces
	lettuce juice	3 ounces

Influenza

Call your doctor. Drink fluids.

1.	Carrot juice	6 ounces
	potato juice	6 ounces
	parsley juice	2 ounces
	watercress juice	2 ounces
2.	Carrot juice	8 ounces
	celery juice	8 ounces

3.	Carrot juice	7 ounces
	parsley juice	2 ounces
	spinach juice	3 ounces
	celery juice	4 ounces

4.	Carrot juice	8 ounces
	celery juice	5 ounces
	radish juice	3 ounces

Insomnia

1.	Carrot juice	10 ounces
	spinach juice	6 ounces

2.	Carrot juice	9 ounces
	celery juice	7 ounces

Kidney problems
Call your doctor.

1.	Celery juice	6 ounces
	beet juice	6 ounces
	cucumber juice	4 ounces

2.	Carrot juice	8 ounces
	beet juice	4 ounces
	celery juice	4 ounces

3.	Dandelion juice	2 ounces
	watercress juice	2 ounces
	lettuce juice	4 ounces
	carrot juice	8 ounces

4.	Cranberry juice	8 ounces
	blueberry juice	4 ounces
	watermelon juice	4 ounces

Laryngitis
Don't talk, drink juice

1.	Pineapple juice	8 ounces
	carrot juice	8 ounces
2.	Pineapple juice	6 ounces
3.	Carrot juice	10 ounces
	spinach juice	6 ounces
4.	Carrot juice	10 ounces
	cucumber juice	3 ounces
	beet juice	3 ounces
5.	Apple juice	8 ounces
	carrot juice	8 ounces

Liver problems

1.	Apple juice	16 ounces
2.	Carrot juice	8 ounces
	celery juice	8 ounces
3.	Carrot juice	10 ounces
	beet juice	4 ounces
	coconut milk	2 ounces
5.	Asparagus juice	4 ounces
	dandelion juice	4 ounces
	carrot juice	8 ounces

Menstruation (excessive)
You may require organic iron.

1.	Fennel juice	8 ounces
	beet juice	8 ounces

2.	Carrot juice celery juice spinach juice	8 ounces 4 ounces 4 ounces
3.	Beet juice nettle juice carrot juice	4 ounces 4 ounces 8 ounces
4.	Carrot juice fennel juice	10 ounces 6 ounces
5.	Cabbage juice lettuce juice carrot juice	4 ounces 4 ounces 8 ounces
6.	Beet greens juice Swiss chard juice carrot juice This combination offers the most organic iron per glass.	4 ounces 4 ounces 8 ounces

Menstruation (irregular)

1.	Parsley juice watercress juice carrot juice apple juice	3 ounces 3 ounces 4 ounces 4 ounces
2.	Fennel juice fig juice parsley juice	6 ounces 6 ounces 4 ounces

Menopausal problems

1.	Carrot juice beet juice pomegranate juice	8 ounces 4 ounces 4 ounces

2.	Carrot juice	8 ounces
	spinach juice	8 ounces
3.	Parsley juice	2 ounces
	celery juice	4 ounces
	carrot juice	7 ounces
	spinach juice	3 ounces
4.	Carrot juice	6 ounces
	turnip juice	3 ounces
	beet juice	3 ounces
	lettuce juice	4 ounces

Mucous membrane, dry

1.	Carrot juice	8 ounces
	celery juice	8 ounces
2.	Carrot juice	8 ounces
	pineapple juice	4 ounces
	papaya juice	4 ounces
3.	Carrot juice	5 ounces
	beet juice	5 ounces
	cucumber juice	5 ounces
	lemon juice	1 ounce

Nervousness

1.	Dandelion juice	6 ounces
	nettle juice	6 ounces
	carrot juice	4 ounces
2.	Brussels sprout juice	4 ounces
	string bean juice	5 ounces
	carrot juice	7 ounces

3.	Beet juice	3 ounces
	cucumber juice	3 ounces
	carrot juice	10 ounces
4.	Celery greens juice	3 ounces
	celery juice	3 ounces
	carrot juice	10 ounces

Neuralgia

1.	Carrot juice	10 ounces
	spinach juice	6 ounces
2.	Carrot juice	10 ounces
	celery juice	6 ounces

Peptic, duodenal or gastric ulcers

See your doctor and try juice therapy.

1.	Cabbage juice	8 ounces
	carrot juice	8 ounces
2.	Potato juice	16 ounces
3.	Pineapple juice	8 ounces
	papaya juice	8 ounces

Prostate problems

See your doctor. Some nutritionists recommend the use of zinc and pumpkin seed oil plus juices.

1.	Lettuce juice	5 ounces
	asparagus juice	5 ounces
	carrot juice	6 ounces

2.	Carrot juice	8 ounces
	beet juice	4 ounces
	cucumber juice	4 ounces
3.	Spinach juice	8 ounces
	carrot juice	8 ounces
4.	Cranberry juice	8 ounces
	blueberry juice	8 ounces

Psoriasis

1.	Carrot juice	10 ounces
	beet juice	3 ounces
	cucumber juice	3 ounces
2.	Carrot juice	10 ounces
	spinach juice	6 ounces
3.	Carrot juice	7 ounces
	celery juice	4 ounces
	parsley juice	2 ounces
	spinach juice	3 ounces

Pyorrhea

1.	Orange juice	8 ounces
	grapefruit juice	8 ounces
2.	Orange juice	7 ounces
	grapefruit juice	7 ounces
	lemon juice	2 ounces
3.	Carrot juice	12 ounces
	potato juice	4 ounces
4.	Carrot juice	10 ounce
	beet juice	3 ounces
	cucumber juice	3 ounces

Rheumatism

1.	Beet juice	8 ounces
	watercress juice	4 ounces
	cucumber juice	4 ounces
2.	Celery juice	5 ounces
	cucumber juice	5 ounces
	carrot juice	6 ounces
3.	Cherry juice	16 ounces in divided doses
4.	Spinach juice	8 ounces
	carrot juice	8 ounces

Rhinitis

1.	Carrot juice	9 ounces
	celery juice	5 ounces
	parsley juice	2 ounces
2.	Orange juice	16 ounces
3.	Grapefruit juice	16 ounces
4.	Horseradish, grated	2 ounces
	lemon juice	2 ounces
	water	12 ounces
5.	Pineapple juice	8 ounces
	papaya juice	8 ounces

Sexual drive, weakened

Nutritionists recommend vitamin E, honey and bee pollen. Herbalists say damiana, dong quai and ginseng tea are effective. Aromatherapists laud the essential oils of ylang-ylang and jasmine.

Beet juice	4 ounces
celery juice	4 ounces
carrot juice	8 ounces

Sinus trouble

1.	Lemon juice	2 ounces
	horseradish (grated)	1 ounce
	water	12 ounces
2.	Carrot juice	8 ounces
	beet greens juice	4 ounces
	radish juice	4 ounces
	(with leaves)	
3.	Carrot juice	8 ounces
	papaya juice	8 ounces
4.	Radish juice	2 ounces
	garlic juice	1 ounce
	onion juice	1 ounce
	lemon juice	1 ounce
	water	11 ounces

Skin blemishes

1.	Apple juice	16 ounces
2.	Beet juice	6 ounces
	carrot juice	10 ounces
3.	Potato juice	10 ounces
	quince juice	2 ounces
	cucumber juice	2 ounces
	carrot juice	2 ounces

4.	Asparagus juice	8 ounces
	dandelion juice	4 ounces
	watercress juice	2 ounces
	carrot juice	2 ounces

| 5. | Prune juice | 4 ounces |
| | carrot juice | 12 ounces |

Varicose veins
See your doctor. If they're caused by constipation, add roughage to your diet.

| 1. | Apple juice | 16 ounce |

2.	Asparagus juice	2 ounces
	potato juice	12 ounces
	carrot juice	2 ounces

3.	Carrot juice	8 ounces
	spinach juice	4 ounces
	turnip juice	2 ounces
	watercress juice	2 ounces

Water retention
Herbalists recommend buchu.

| 1. | Asparagus juice | 6 ounces |

| 2. | Dandelion juice | 10 ounces |
| | celery juice | 6 ounces |

3.	Nettle juice	4 ounces
	cucumber juice	4 ounces
	watermelon juice	2 ounces
	carrot juice	6 ounces

| 4. | Cucumber juice | 8 ounces |
| | celery juice | 8 ounces |

5 Juices for Cleansing
...Juices for Healing

In general, fruit juices are cleansing, while the raw juices from vegetables are healing and restorative. After an illness, the body has to "take out the garbage." There's a lot of toxic material and waste products, dead white blood cells, killed viruses and bacteria, and loads of unspeakable glop that you have to get rid of. Fruit juices are wonderful for detoxifying the body and helping to carry out excess waste. Then a combination of raw fruit juices and vegetable juices can help restore your body to a healthful condition.

Some raw fruit juices are better cleansers in certain conditions than others, and some raw vegetable juices are faster restoratives in specific conditions than other juices. The following list contains those raw juices considered by nutritionists to be the most effective for cleansing and restoring in particular circumstances.

FRUIT JUICES ARE WONDERFUL FOR DETOXIFYING THE BODY AND CARRYING OUT WASTE.

Once health is restored, all raw fruit juices and all raw vegetable juices should be used freely, depending on the availability of the produce. The listings are not to be used in place of the advice of a health professional but in conjunction with professional treatment or advice

Raw Fruit Juices for Cleansing and Detoxification

SITUATION	SUGGESTED JUICES
Acne	papaya, strawberry, blueberry
Anemia	prune, cherry, grape, citrus fruits
Arthritis	Watermelon, cherry, apple, prune
Bladder problems	Cranberry, blueberry, pear, watermelon
Bruises	Papaya, pineapple, grapefruit, orange, lemon, lime
Cancer	Grape, citrus fruits
Colds-and flu	Pineapple, papaya, all citrus fruits
Constipation	Prune, watermelon, papaya, pear, peach, melon, lemon, lime, strawberry, quince, apple

Situation	Suggested Juices
Cough	All citrus juices, papaya
Cramps	Cherry, black cherry, watermelon
Diarrhea	Cranberry, blueberry
Ear problems	All citrus juices
Fever	Cranberry, blueberry, strawberry, all citrus juices
Fluid retention	Cranberry, blueberry, strawberry, watermelon
Gall bladder problems	Cherry
Gout	Pineapple, papaya, apple, grape, strawberry, citrus fruits
Hemorrhoids	Prune, grape
Indigestion	Papaya, strawberry, cranberry, peach, pineapple, apple, all citrus juices if tolerated
Kidney problems	Watermelon, papaya, pineapple, cranberry, blueberry, grape, all melons
Liver problems	Papaya, pear, apple, all citrus juices
Prostate problems	Cherry, cranberry, blueberry, pear, strawberry, watermelon
Pyorrhea	All citrus juices, pineapple, strawberry
Rheumatism	Apple, cherry, black cherry, strawberry, all citrus juices
Sciatica	Pineapple, cherry, papaya

Situation	Suggested Juices
Skin problems	Watermelon, cranberry, grape, blueberry, melon, citrus juices
Sore throat	Pineapple, all citrus juices, papaya
Ulcers	Papaya
Urinary tract problems	Cranberry, blueberry, grapefruit, watermelon
Varicose veins	Grapefruit, watermelon

Raw Vegetable Juices for Cleansing and Detoxification

Situation	Suggested Juices
Acne	Carrot, cucumber, dandelion, endive, parsnip, spinach, lettuce, asparagus
Anemia	Asparagus, beet, dandelion, endive, kale, lettuce, parsley, spinach, carrot, turnip, watercress
Arthritis	Carrot, cucumber, spinach, parsley, beet, radish, turnip
Asthma	Cabbage, carrot, celery, kale, potato, watercress
Bladder problems	Carrot, beet, cucumber, dandelion, endive, parsley, tomato, turnip, squash
Blood pressure problems	Beet, cabbage, cucumber, spinach, garlic

Juices for Cleansing

Situation	Suggested Juices
Bronchitis	Horseradish, garlic, cabbage, celery, turnip, beet
Cancer	Carrot, asparagus, beet, parsley, kale, turnip, Swiss chard
Colitis	Cabbage, spinach, beet, spinach
Constipation	Cabbage, celery, endive, potato, cucumber
Cough	Onion, scallion, horseradish
Diabetes	Brussels sprout, string bean, carrot, lettuce, celery, parsley
Diarrhea	Carrot, celery, spinach, parsley, beet
Eczema	Cucumber, radish, carrot, spinach, potato, beet, papaya, nettle
Eyes	Asparagus, beet, carrot, celery, dandelion, endive, parsley, pepper, turnip
Fever	Cabbage, onion, garlic, cucumber
Fluid retention	Cucumber, celery
Gout	Asparagus, string bean, carrot, celery, parsley, spinach, fennel, tomato
Hay fever	Carrot, kale, parsnip
Hemorrhoids	Carrot, potato, watercress, spinach, nettle, turnip
Hair loss	Alfalfa, cabbage, cucumber, spinach, lettuce, pepper, watercress

Juices for Cleansing

SITUATION	SUGGESTED JUICES
Insomnia	Lettuce, celery
Jaundice	Beet
Kidney problems	Carrot, celery, beet, asparagus, cabbage, cucumber
Laryngitis	Cucumber, carrot, spinach, beet
Liver problems	Asparagus, beet, dandelion, carrot, celery, endive, kale, lettuce, parsnip, spinach, tomato, watercress
Menopause	Carrot, beet, pomegranate, spinach, parsley, turnip, beet, Swiss chard
Nervousness	Carrot, dandelion, nettle, asparagus, celery, fennel, lettuce, spinach, beet, Brussels sprout
Prostate problems	Asparagus, carrot, lettuce, parsley, spinach, cucumber, beet
Psoriasis	Cucumber
Pyorrhea	Cabbage, kale, spinach
Rheumatism	Beet, watercress, cucumber, asparagus, celery, carrot
Sinus problems	Horseradish, radish, carrot, garlic, onion
Ulcers	Cabbage, carrot, potato, parsnip, spinach
Varicose veins (from constipation) watercress	Asparagus, potato, carrot spinach, turnip.

6
Buying a Juicer
Your Home Juice Bar

You can squeeze an orange by hand, but it's more difficult to squeeze a carrot and get juice from it. So, since carrots are among the most valuable sources of raw juice, you're going to have to buy a juicer.

Juicers come in a variety of price ranges and are made by a number of companies. Some are noisier than others. Some vibrate more and extract less of the juice. Most are fairly easy to maintain and assemble for use. I'll discuss the different types of machines, then list a variety of juicers with their features and suggested list prices. This listing is not a recommendation, and is by no means complete, but is offered as information only. In choosing a juicer, you should consider your needs and what you

🍂
YOU CAN'T HAND-SQUEEZE JUICE FROM A CARROT—SO YOU'RE GOING TO HAVE TO BUY A JUICER.

can afford, and check out as many juicers as you can before making your purchase.

Juicers are not blenders.

What comes out of a juicer and what comes out of a blender are not the same. Juicers deliver the juice and leave the pulp behind.

A blender chops up whatever is put into it and turns it into a liquid—maybe a mushy liquid, but a liquid nevertheless. It combines the liquid and the pulp. Blenders cannot deliver pure juice, which can become body-active in 15 minutes. Blended material requires a much longer digestion and assimilation time.

> HAND JUICERS CAN SERVE FOR ORANGE OR GRAPEFRUIT BUT ARE USELESS WHEN IT COMES TO APPLES, BEETS, CARROTS, CELERY AND SO ON. YOU NEED A HIGH-SPEED ELECTRIC JUICER TO CONVERT MOST FRUITS AND VEGETABLES INTO JUICE.

But blenders can be valuable and lucky is the person who owns both. If you do, you can liquefy a banana, mix it with peach and orange juice and really fortify your body.

KINDS OF JUICERS

There are two basic types of juicers outside of the conventional hand-operated juicers we are accustomed to. Hand juicers can serve for oranges or grapefruit but are useless when it comes to apples, beets, carrots, celery and so on. You have to have a high-speed electric juicer to convert most fruits and vegetables into raw juice. The two basic types are as follows:

Centrifugal Juicer

This juicer chops up the fruit or vegetable in a plastic or stainless steel basket, then spins the contents at very high speed to separate the juice from the pulp. The juice comes out of a spigot and the pulp remains behind to be removed afterward.

There is a version of the centrifugal juicer that includes a *pulp ejector*: the action is the same, but there is an additional delivery area that automatically ejects the pulp. Its value is that you can make more juice without having to stop and remove the accumulated pulp. If you have a large family and have to make large amounts of juice, this may be an advantage. However, it has been my experience that it also may leave some of the juice in the pulp. You have to balance the options between the amount of juice you need at one sitting and the possible loss of some of the juice with the pulp. You'll get good juice from both of these juicers.

Masticating Juicer

This juicer grinds the fruit or vegetable into a paste before spinning at high speed to squeeze the juice through a screen set into the juicer bottom.

CENTRIFUGAL (EXTRACTION) JUICERS

Acme Juicerator, Models 5001, 6001, 7001

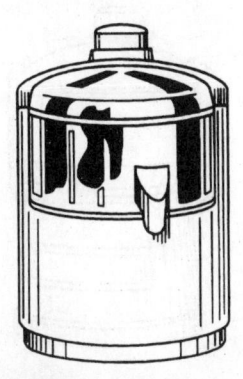

Stainless steel basket/spinner and blades, 3600 rpm, "no-maintenance" brushless motor, self-adjusting clutch, 2-quart capacity centrifugal chamber. Optional citrus attachment for all models steps motor down to 300 rpm; 10-year limited warranty Models 6001 and 7001, 5 years on 5001. Suggested retail, 5001, $206; 6001, $299; 7001, $255. Acme Juicer Mfg. Co., Waring Products Div. D.C.A., 283 Main Street, New Hartford, CT 06507, 203 379-0731.

Similar models are available under the name Waring Professional.

Miracle Juicer, MJ 1000

One-piece stainless steel cutter/strainer, automatic pulp ejection, external pulp container allows continuous juicing, special hopper for small fruit, high-speed motor claimed to produce drier pulp and therefore more juice; 1-year guarantee. Suggested retail $124.95. Distributed by Miracle Exclusives, Inc., 3 Elm Street, Locust Valley, NY 11560, 1-800 645-6360.

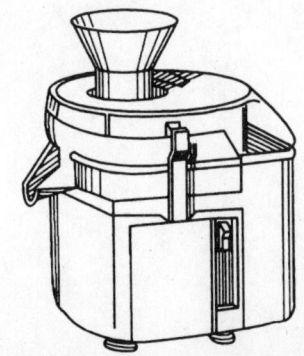

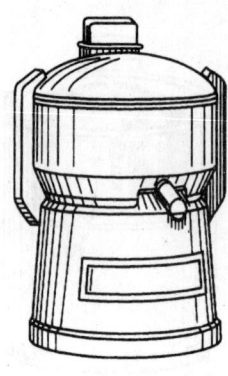

Omega Juicer

Stainless steel construction, claims "ultra-quiet" operation. Optional citrus attachment gears machine down from 3600 rpm to 250, allowing "hand" juicing of oranges, lemons, etc. Ten-year guarantee against defects in material and workmanship. Suggested retail $234. Omega Inc., 291 Lyters Lane, Harrisburg, PA 17111, 1-800 633-3401.

Perfect Juicer, MJ 600

Pulp ejector, one-piece stainless steel cutter/strainer, 2 speeds; model 606 includes blender and grinder attachments; 1-year guarantee. Suggested retail MJ600, $114.95; MJ606, $139.95. Miracle Exclusives, Inc. (see above for address).

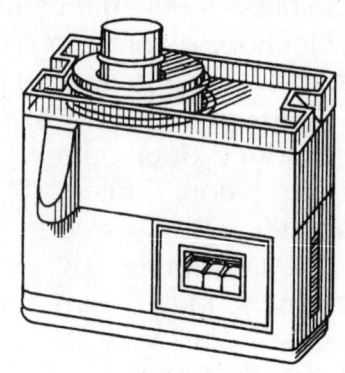

Phoenix Juicer

Two speeds, automatic pulp ejector. Stainless steel blade and spinner, filling tray for small fruit (e.g. berries), hidden cord, safety lock, .27 hp motor operating at 11,000 rpm, 5-year guarantee on parts and labor. Suggested retail $169.95. Phoenix Housewares Corporation, PO Box 451, Fresh Meadows, NY 11365.

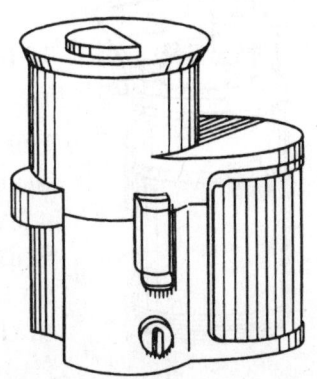

Singer Juice Giant
Juice Extractor, Model 774

Stainless steel grater and spinner, separate containers keep pulp and juice apart. Interior cord storage, safety interlock switch, 1-year warranty. Suggested retail $64.95 Singer Sewing Company, 200 Metroplex Drive, Edison NJ 08818, 1-800 877-7391

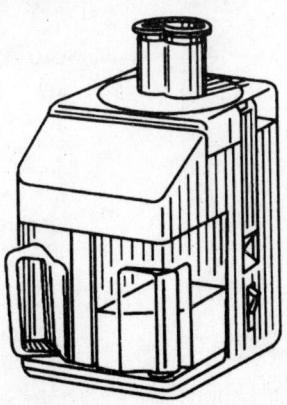

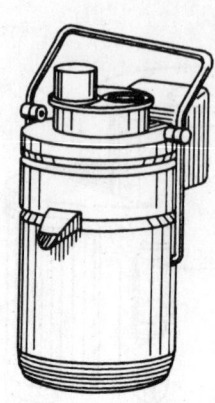

Ultra-Matic MJ 700

Stainless steel cutting disc, strainer basket, juice bowl and juicer body, automatic outside pulp ejection. 45-watt motor; 1-year guarantee. Suggested retail $299. Miracle Exclusives, Inc. (see above for address and phone).

Waring Juice Extractor, JE 504-1

Stainless steel strainer and shredder/blade, 6-cup capacity pulp collector twists off for cleaning; 5-year warranty on motor, 1 year on other components. Suggested retail, $74.95. Waring Products Division, Dynamics Corporation of America, 283 Main Street, New Hartford, CT 06057, 203 379-0731.

MASTICATION JUICER
Champion Juicer

Rotating cutter on a shaft is claimed to extract more nutrients from vegetables and juices than other types of juicers. Easily convertible to grater or homogenizer (for preparation of nut butters, ice cream, etc.); grain mill attachment available; 5-year guarantee. Suggested retail $270. Platasket Manufacturing Co., Inc., Lodi, CA; distributed by Quality Health Products, Inc., 922 Black Diamond Way, Lodi, CA 95240.

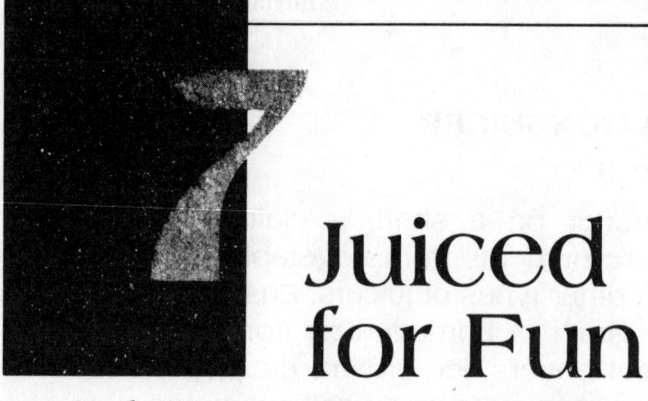

Juiced for Fun
Drinking Your Health

Not everything has to be serious. Nobody likes a bore.

If you can't have fun with your juicer, it can get to be a nag.

This is the part of the book where the juicer and its cousin the blender combine their talents.

We're going to make beverages that taste good, are fun to drink, can be served at parties—and will be healthful, too.

Fresh juices whenever possible, frozen juices if you can't get fresh, but never canned juices.

❧ Strawberry Shake
    1 cup fresh strawberries
    1 cup fresh orange juice
    1 tablespoon honey

Blend well and serve over an ice cube. Loaded with vitamin C and carotenes.

❧ Pineapple/Carrot Surprise

    2 cups fresh pineapple juice
    juice from 2 or 3 carrots
    1 ounce lemon juice

Blend well and serve. The combination of the acid fruit and the carrot goes particularly well and is very stimulating.

❧ Orange Punch

    3 cups orange juice
    2 cups apricot juice
    4 tablespoons lemon juice
    1 cup grapefruit juice

Mix them all together, add honey if you need to sweeten it, add ice in the summer time. Serves 6.

❧ Grape Delight

    3 cups grape juice
    2 cups pineapple juice
    1 cup pear juice
    1 cup celery juice
    3 tablespoons lemon juice

Combine the juices and serve in chilled glasses. Serves 6.

> IF YOU CAN'T HAVE FUN WITH YOUR JUICER, IT CAN GET TO BE A NAG.

❧ Skin and Hair Beauty Cocktail

Put into your juicer equal portions of apples, pears, carrots, celery, lettuce and spinach. Turn on the juicer and put your glass under the spout for a glass of beautifying vitamins and minerals.

❧ Cranberry Cocktail

    1 pound spray-free cranberries
    1 glass orange juice

1 glass apple juice
2 teaspoons lemon juice

Mix the juices together. Add honey if the cranberries are too bitter.

🌢 Special Lemonade

1 pound of cherries, juiced
6 lemons, juiced
5 apricots, juiced
$1/4$ cup strawberry juice

Mix well and dilute with 5 glasses ice water.

🌢 Appetite Builder

3 cups sauerkraut juice
2 teaspoons parsley juice
2 tablespoons beet juice
2 tablespoons spinach juice

Mix well and drink half an hour before mealtime. The tangy taste will stimulate even the most stubborn appetite. Try it!

🌢 Blood-Builder

Use this mixture as a beverage before and during meals. Eliminates the desire for coffee and builds red blood.

$1/2$ cup carrot juice
$1/2$ cup spinach juice
$1/2$ cup beet juice
$1/2$ cup mustard greens juice
$1/4$ cup coconut milk

🌢
BEET AND MUSTARD GREENS JUICES PROMOTE BLOOD HEALTH.

❧ Morning Nose Clearer
If you get up with a stuffed nose, forget orange juice and try this mixture instead.
   3/4 cup carrot juice
   2 tablespoons radish juice
   2 tablespoons horseradish juice
   1 teaspoon lemon juice
Mix well and sip slowly.

❧ Health Shake
   1/4 cup strawberry juice
   1/4 cup orange juice
   1/4 cup pineapple juice
   1/4 cup coconut milk
Amounts do not have to be precise. Mix and really enjoy what you are drinking.

❧ Vitamin C and the Bioflavonoids
Sounds like a rock group but really provides help for vitamin-hungry circulatory systems.
   1/2 glass orange juice
   1/2 glass grapefruit juice
   1/2 lemon, juiced
Mix and drink.

❧ Potassium Broth
This mixture is heavy with minerals, particularly potassium, which is difficult to obtain from regular diets.
   1/2 cup carrot juice
   1/4 cup celery juice
   2 tablespoons spinach juice
   2 tablespoons lettuce juice
   2 tablespoons parsley juice
The quantities don't have to be exact, so put the various vegetables in your juicer and turn it on. Drink whatever gets into your glass.

❧ Midmorning or Afternoon Energy Booster

    3 teaspoons parsley juice
    2 teaspoons watercress juice
    1/2 cup carrot juice
    1/2 cup celery juice

Try this instead of coffee and Danish pastry during your coffee break.

❧ Fresh Tomato Juice

    1 cup tomato juice
    2 tablespoons celery juice
    1 teaspoon lemon juice

Mix and serve.

❧ Rhubarb Atom Bomb

Constipation trouble gives way to this mixture for a good morning.

    3/4 cup rhubarb juice
    1/4 cup apple juice

For soothing and natural but effective action on stubborn bowels.

❧ Fresh Fruit Soup

A surprising taste for those who need soup but don't like soup. Even the kids will ask for more.

    1 1/2 cups strawberry juice
    1 1/2 cups pineapple juice
    1/2 cup cherry juice
    1 cup carrot juice
    1/4 cup tomato juice

After juicing and mixing, add 2 teaspoons of lemon juice. If you like, garnish with a tablespoon or two of yogurt.

❧ Cranberry-Grapefruit Mix

Wash the cranberries in hot water and pick out those that don't look so good. Peel the grapefruit and scrape off the white stuff that clings to the inside peel (rich in bioflavonoids) and put that in the juicer as well.

    1 grapefruit, juiced
    1/2 cup cranberries, juiced
    1 1/2 cup water
    1 tablespoon honey

❧ Yogurt-Tomato Surprise

If the kids won't drink juice, let them try this. After you taste it there may not be any left for them!

    2 cups fresh tomato juice
    1 tablespoon unflavored yogurt
    1/2 teaspoon lemon juice
    1/4 teaspoon white horseradish (start with a little less)
    1/4 teaspoon honey
    dash of sea salt

Blend well and serve over an ice cube.

❧
A SURPRISE TASTE TREAT FOR KIDS!

❧ Winter's Day Mulled Apple Juice

Make 2 quarts of fresh apple juice if there's a crowd in the house. Put the juice in a pot and add:

    1 1-inch stick of cinnamon
    1/4 teaspoon nutmeg
    1/4 teaspoon allspice
    6 whole cloves
    1/2 cup honey

Simmer slowly for twenty minutes. Remove the cloves if they haven't completely dissolved, and serve in mugs topped with a slice of fresh orange. Wait for the applause!

🌿 Mystery Drink

The one who guesses the formula gets another cup.

    8 large carrots, juiced
    2 large cucumbers, juiced
    8 ounces coconut milk

Blend to a froth and serve at once.

🌿 Pick-Me-Up

    1 papaya, juiced
    1 orange, juiced
    1 carrot, juiced
    $1/2$ cup unflavored yogurt

Blend well; add 1/2 cup more orange juice and some ice; blend at high speed.

🌿 Carrot-Apple

    $1 1/2$ cups carrot juice
    $1/2$ cup apple juice
    $1/2$ teaspoon honey
    dash of cloves

Blend to a froth. Delicious and a mild laxative as well.

🌿 Orange Nectar

    $1/2$ cup juice from fresh orange
    Put in the blender with two soft bananas
    2 tablespoons of honey
    $1/4$ teaspoon almond extract
    1 quart milk

Blend until frothy, then serve. If you have a skinny child who won't drink milk and you're worried about his bones and teeth, make this concoction and stop worrying.

❧ Watermelon-ade
Puree 2 cups of ripe watermelon. Put in a blender with
    1/2 cup lemon juice
    1/2 teaspoon grated lemon rind
    1 tablespoon honey
    2 cups water
Blend until the honey is well mixed.

❧ Hot-Day Pickup
    1/2 cup orange juice
    1/2 cup apple juice
    1 teaspoon lime juice
In a tall glass over ice, this is cooling and tasty.

❧ Cantaloupe Milk Shake
    1/2 cup milk
    2 tablespoons lemon juice
    1 tablespoon honey
    flesh of 1 ripe cantaloupe
Blend till frothy, serve over ice.

❧ Banana Flip
    1 large banana
    1 tablespoon honey
    1/8 teaspoon almond extract
    1/2 teaspoon grated orange rind
    1 1/2 cups ice-cold milk
Blend at high speed and serve over ice.

❧ Honey/Fruit Punch
    1 cup orange juice
    1 teaspoon lemon juice
    1/2 cup pineapple juice
    2 cups water

1 teaspoon honey
Mix, chill and serve.

❧ Golden Drink
Tastes a lot better than it reads.
1 beet root, juiced
5 leaves Romaine lettuce, juiced
½ orange
3 carrots
Mix and drink.

❧ Summer Cleanser
4 ounces pineapple juice
2 ounces orange juice
1 ounce papaya juice
1 ounce carrot juice
a little lime juice
Put in a tall glass and sip.

❧ South Seas
Put all these in the blender:
1 small apple, unpeeled but cored and quartered
½ cup fresh orange or grapefruit juice
1 cup fresh papaya
2 teaspoons of peanut butter (yes, peanut butter!)
Blend until smooth, then serve.

PEANUT BUTTER ADDS A TROPICAL TOUCH.

❧ Apple Swinger
½ cup apple juice
¼ cup celery leaves
2 teaspoons lemon juice
½ cup cracked ice
Blend well.

❧ Pear Cooler

When pears are in season, core two pears and cut in half, then dice and put them in the blender. Add the juice from three apricots and:
- $1/4$ cup lemon juice
- 1 tablespoon crushed ice
- 1 tablespoon honey

Blend well till smooth.

❧ Thirst Quencher

- 1 cup apple juice
- 1 cup orange juice
- $1/2$ carrot, minced
- 1 rib of celery
- $1/2$ banana
- 2 green leaves spinach or Romaine lettuce
- 1 teaspoon crushed almonds
- 1 teaspoon raisins
- 2 sprigs parsley

Blend well until all is liquefied, then add crushed ice and blend again.

❧ Sexy Vegetable Juice

Place in the blender:
- 2 tomatoes
- 1 pepper
- 1 carrot and its top
- 2 onions
- 1 cabbage leaf

Blend for two minutes.

❧ Apple Swinger

- $1/2$ cup apple juice
- $1/4$ cup celery leaves

2 teaspoons lemon juice
   ½ cup cracked ice
Blend well.

❧ Thick Shake
   1 cup skim milk
   ½ cup of any fruit juice
   ½ teaspoon vanilla extract
   3 ice cubes
Blend to a froth.

❧ Waist Watcher
   ¼ cup cold skim milk
   ½ cup blueberries
   1 teaspoon vanilla
Blend to a froth and add an ice cube if you like it cold.

❧ Milk of the Lion
For pure energy:
   2 tablespoons dry milk powder
   ½ cup cold skim milk
   1 tablespoon tahini paste
   2 tablespoons of any soft nut
   ½ cup of any fresh fruit
Blend till foamy, then drink.

❧ Green Magic
In the juicer:
   1 carrot
   1 cucumber
   3 fistfuls of spinach
Juice and serve.

❧ Strawberry Bobby
In the juicer:
- 1 medium apple
- 2 wedges of pineapple
- 1 cup strawberries (remove the green tops)

Juice and drink.

❧ Orange Genie
In the juicer:
- $1/2$ papaya, peeled and pitted
- 1 medium peach, pitted
- $1/2$ grapefruit

Juice and enjoy.

❧ Banana Floozie
Simmer a teaspoonful of marjoram in a cup of water for five minutes. Cool and put the solution into a blender with:
- 1 cup banana juice
- 1 egg white
- crushed ice

Blend until frothy and serve. (You can use pineapple juice instead of banana juice.)

❧ Apple-Ap
- $1/2$ cup dried apricots
- 1 cup apple juice

Blend and enjoy.

❧ Apple-Ginger
- 1 cup apple juice
- $1/2$ cup cherry juice
- small piece of ginger
- crushed ice

Blend and drink.

❧ Plum Delight
3 plums, stones removed
1/2 cup plum juice
1 cup apple juice
crushed ice
Blend and drink.

❧ Pine-Grape
In a blender:
    chunk of pineapple
    1 cup grape juice
    crushed ice
Blend with a teaspoon of honey

❧ Before-Dinner Aperitif
    1 cup tomato juice
    1 cup celery juice
    few sprigs of parsley
    juice of 1/2 lemon
    1 cup carrot juice
    crushed ice
    sprinkle of sea salt
Drinks for four.

Mix and Juice

❧ A couple of apples and a handful of pitted cherries.

❧ A couple of apples and a small bunch of grapes. Remove grapes from the stem and wash thoroughly first.

❧ A pear, a peach, as many cherries as you have. Wash thoroughly and juice.

- Apples and pears. Wash thoroughly first.

- Two apples, a handful of strawberries, a squeeze of lemon. Pluck out or cut off the strawberry greens after washing and throw them away. There's no nutritional value to them.

- A couple of handfuls of cranberries, a couple of apples. Wash very well before juicing. Cranberries are very bitter but the apple juice is sweet. Makes a wonderful drink and helps protect the genitourinary system against infection. Good for men as well as for women.

- A couple of handfuls of cranberries, a grapefruit, an orange. This mixture is even more acid than the cranberry/apple one, so you may want to add a little honey. Taste it first.

- One papaya—peeled and pit removed—a large bunch of grapes—any variety—a squeeze of lemon juice. Remove grapes from stem and wash well in a strainer. Juice the mixture.

- Half a ripe papaya—peeled and pit removed—a peach—pit removed—half a grapefruit, pink or white. Wash thoroughly before juicing.

- A chunk of pineapple without the peel, a handful of strawberries, a ripe apple. Wash fruits, remove green from strawberries.

🍀 This mixture requires the use of a blender. Juice a ripe apple and a ripe pear and put the juice in a blender with a cup of water and half a dozen pitted prunes. Blend at high speed then drink. A good drink to keep you regular. Even kids will drink it.

🍀 A cup each of honeydew and cantaloupe flesh. Juice with a cup of watermelon fruit. Turn on juicer and collect the juice. Then put the watermelon rind, cut in small pieces, into juicer and juice it; mix all the juices and enjoy.

🍀 If you are retaining water, juice a chunk of watermelon including rind and seeds, and drink.

🍀 Stomach a little queasy? Try a couple of apples and a teaspoonful of grated ginger root. Juice together and sip slowly.

🍀 You can please your sweet tooth and still save calories when you combine the talents of your freezer and your juicer. Freeze a banana and some strawberries (after washing and removing the green tops). Juice two oranges and put the juice in a blender with the frozen fruit. Blend at medium speed for just one minute and serve like ice cream.

WHAT TO DO WITH THE LEFTOVER PULP

There are many ways to utilize the pulp left over from juicing to enrich and flavor other foods. The important thing is to use it promptly or to freeze it in small quantities for future use. Whatever you can't consume can be a valuable addition to your compost heap—providing nutrients for future vegetables and fruits!

Fruit Pulp

- Apple, pear, apricot, or peach pulp are wonderful additions to hot cereal. With a few shakes of cinnamon, this breakfast treat will be naturally sweet without added sugar or concentrated sweeteners.

- Fruit pulp can be mixed with yogurt or cottage cheese, or whipped with silken tofu for a very pleasing and healthful snack. If the fruit is tart, a squirt of maple syrup or honey will mellow the flavor. Top with a handful of granola, toasted seeds or nuts, for crunch and fiber.

- If you puree your fruit pulp, add cinnamon or nutmeg, and warm, you have a wonderful topping for pancakes, waffles, french toast, or muffins. Again, sweeten to taste, if necessary.

- A frothy fruit shake can be made by combining milk, plain yogurt, soy milk, or fruit juice with fruit pulp. Add slices of frozen banana for natural sweetening and thickening. Here are two good combinations:

❧ Hawaiian Smoothie

Blend one cup pineapple juice with $1/2$ cup peach pulp. With motor running, add 6 slices of frozen banana, one at a time and blend until smooth.

❧ Very Berry Shake

Blend one cup milk, plain yoghurt, or soy milk with $1/2$ banana and $1/2$ cup berry pulp. With motor running, add 6 frozen strawberries, one at a time and blend until smooth.

Fruit or vegetable pulp is an excellent addition to recipes for muffins, cakes, and breads. Try the following tasty recipes:

❧ Carrot-Pineapple-Coconut Cake

2 cups carrot pulp
$1/2$ cup pineapple pulp
1 cup grated coconut
3 cups flour
1 tablespoon baking soda
1 tablespoon cinnamon
$1/2$ teaspoon nutmeg
1 cup honey
4 eggs
1 cup canola oil
1 tablespoon vanilla
$1 1/2$ cups nuts

Mix the pulps together, add the honey, oil and vanilla and blend well. Sift dry ingredients and add coconut and nuts. Pour in prepared pan. Bake at 350° for 50-60 minutes. Also for muffins. Fill muffin pan 3/4 full and bake 40-45 minutes.

❧ Squash Bread

1 1/2 cups yellow squash pulp
2 cups flour
1/2 teaspoon baking soda
1 teaspoon baking powder
2 1/2 teaspoons vanilla
2 teaspoons cinammon
1 1/2 cups mashed dates
2 eggs
1/2 cup canola oil
optional: 1 cup nuts

Beat squash with date mash. Add oil slowly and mix well. Add eggs and vanilla and beat. Sift all dry ingredients together and add all at once to squash mixture. Beat until blended. Stir in nuts. Pour in prepared 5" x 9" pan. Bake at 350° for one hour. Insert toothpick in center. Bread is done if it comes out clean.

❧ Chick Pea Carrot Loaf

1 box Near East falafel mix
1 cup carrot pulp
8 ounces water
4 tablespoons tomato sauce

Oil or butter 5" x 7" x 2" loaf pan. In a bowl mix all of the ingredients. Put into oiled pan and bake at 310° for ten minutes before cutting. Serve with cucumber dressing or tahini sauce.

The following carrot pulp recipes were created by Georgia Ray's Organic Gourmet Caterers of Greenwich, Connecticut.

❧ Jalapeño Carrot Corn Pudding
1 large can creamed corn
1 cup corn kernels (fresh or frozen)
$1/2$ pound carrot pulp
$1/2$ cup each chopped onion, celery, and green pepper
2 cloves garlic
$1/4$ cup chopped scallions
$1/4$ cup chopped parsley
3 eggs
1 tablespoon arrowroot or flour
1 cup milk or soymilk
2 tablespoons chopped chili peppers
$1 1/2$ tablespoons honey

Preheat oven to 350°. Sauté onions, celery, and green pepper in 1 tablespoon of olive oil until tender. Add the carrot pulp and cook for a few minutes longer. Mix eggs, milk, and honey together. Add the hot cooked vegetables slowly to the batter. Mix well and pour into a greased casserole dish and bake for 1 to $1 1/2$ hours or until set.

Optional: Top with soy cheese or Parmesan cheese and/or toasted cashews. Serve with sliced tomato-cucumber salad with parsley and mild vinaigrette.

❧ Lentil Polenta Patties

1 pound red lentils
$1/2$ pound carrot pulp
$1/2$ pound cooked polenta
$1/2$ pound cooked millet
3 stalks celery, chopped fine
1 large onion, chopped fine
1 teaspoon saffron
$1/2$ teaspoon ground black pepper
$1/4$ teaspoon cayenne pepper
$1/4$ cup rice vinegar
$1/4$ teaspoon thyme
2 cloves garlic, minced
soy sauce and Dijon mustard, to taste

Soak lentils for 3 hours in water. Drain and rinse lentils. Cook in just enough water to cover for 5-10 minutes, or until tender. Drain excess water into carrot pulp, and steam 5 minutes. Meanwhile sauté celery, onions and garlic in 1 tablespoon of olive or canola oil. Add all ingredients to a large bowl and mix thoroughly. Season to your taste with salt, soy sauce, and Dijon mustard. Form into patties and chill.

Sauté in canola or olive oil on one side until brown. Flip and put in 350° oven for ten minutes longer. A cast iron skillet works well.

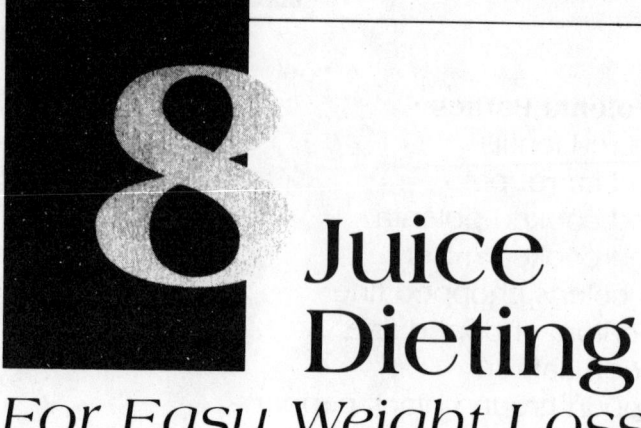

8 Juice Dieting
For Easy Weight Loss

When most people diet they get irritable, anxious, overtired and just plain nasty. One of the reasons is that they are not taking in enough nutrients to keep their body happy while they try to burn off excess fat.

A water fast will result in weight loss. No doubt about it. But, a water fast can be dangerous. In fact, the following conditions preclude any kind of fasting:

tumors	bleeding ulcers
cerebral disease	kidney disease
gout	liver disease
blood disease	recent heart trouble
active lung disease	diabetes

Seniors should not fast without advice from their doctors.

Juice fasting, provided you are in normal

health, can be the easiest and most comfortable way to lose a few pounds.

Juice fasting provides the highest density of nutrients for the calorie intake.

In other words, you get the most nutrition and the least fat during a juice fast.

Let's look at what you get when you juice a half pound of carrots. Your glass will contain, approximately, these nutrients:

calories	78
protein	2 grams
carbohydrate	18 grams
calcium	69 milligrams
phosphorus	67 milligrams
iron	1.3 milligrams
sodium	88 milligrams
potassium	635 milligrams
vitamin A	20,460 milligrams
vitamin C	15 milligrams
vitamin B:	
thiamine	.11 milligrams
riboflavin	.10 milligrams
niacin	1.1 milligrams

No cholesterol, no triglycerides, no fat. If you substitute a glass of juice for one of your meals, let's say lunch, and eat your regular breakfast and dinner, you will lose about 8 to 10 pounds in a month. Because the natural sugars will be brought to the body tissues and your brain in about fifteen minutest you shouldn't feel anxious or nervous. Two full glasses will still only cost 158 calories. Figure the calories on your average lunch to estimate the savings.

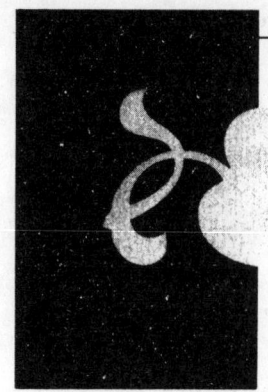

Appendix
Vitamin/Mineral Tables

NOTE:
The symptoms noted could occur only when the daily intake of the vitamins mentioned has been less than the minimum daily requirement over a prolonged period. These non-specific symptoms do not alone prove nutritional deficiency but may be caused by any great number of conditions or may have functional causes. If these symptoms persist they may indicate a condition other than a vitamin or mineral deficiency. It is recommended that any unusual or prolonged symptoms be looked into by a competent professional.

For any treatment of diagnosis of illness see your physician. This chart is not intended to be diagnostic or prescriptive, but is for information purposes only. Individuals allergic to certain dietary supplements should consult a physician for advice.

KEY

IU	International Units (measure of strength)
mg	milligrams (measure of strength)
mcg	micrograms (measure of strength)
RDA	Recommended Daily Allowance
SDR	Supplement Dosage Recommended (SDR): the supplemental dosage recommended is the amount suggested to help prevent or overcome nutritional deficiencies in conjunction with a good diet, exercise, and a healthy lifestyle. Professional supervision recommended.

Supplementation and the inclusion of foods from the food source column is the best way to obtain needed nutrients.

Supplements are best taken with meals. The water soluble vitamins (B-Complex and C) should be taken in divided doses during the day, or in a time released form.

VITAMINS

Nutrients	RDA/SDR Levels	Food Sources
Vitamin A: retinol and beta carotene— most effective with C, D, E, R, B-complex, calcium, phosphorus, zinc	RDA 5000 IU SDR 1000-2500 IU Toxicity 50000 IU Symptoms hair loss No toxicity for beta carotene	Yellow, orange, and dark green vegetables and fruits, liver, lemon grass, eggs, whole milk, fish liver oil capsules, or betacarotene tablets
B-complex: all of the B vitamin family— best to take all B vitamins together	SDR 10-60 mg	Nutritional yeast, liver, whole grains, brown rice, meat, eggs
B-1: thiamine— most effective with C, E, B-2, B-complex, manganese	RDA 1.5 mg SDR 10-60 mg	Whole wheat, brown rice, other whole grains, molasses, raw clams, liver, legumes, nuts, fish, poultry, germ and bran of rice, wheat and corn, nutritional yeast, milk
B-2: riboflavin— most effective with B-complex, B-6, C, niacin	RDA 1.7 mg SDR 10-60 mg	Whole wheat, brown rice, other whole grains, molasses, liver, lean meat, milk, cheese, nutritional yeast, nuts, legumes (peas & beans), bran of rice, wheat & corn, egg yolk, avocado, sunflower and sesame seeds

ANTAGONISTS	BODY PARTS & FUNCTIONS AIDED	DEFICIENCY SYMPTOMS & BENEFICIAL USES
Caffeine, alcohol, mineral oil, excess iron, tobacco, ultraviolet rays	Eyes, health of skin, mucous membranes, hair and bone growth, resistance to infection, teeth, gums, pregnancy & lactation, anti-oxidant	Night blindness, itching eyes, tooth and gum disorders, susceptibility to colds, infections and viruses, sinus and respiratory problems, asthma, bronchitis, allergies, cystitis, dry skin, eczema, acne, psoriasis, blemishes, lack of appetite, fatigue, migraine headaches
Caffeine, alcohol, sugars, tobacco, perspiration	Energy, food, metabolism and digestion, intestinal health, growth, healthy blood formation, muscle maintenance	Stress, nerve disorders, fatigue, headache, hypoglycemia, anemia, allergies, acne, dry skin, insomnia, dry or falling hair, menstrual difficulties, nausea, constipation, digestive problems
Stress, tobacco, caffeine, fever, alcohol, antibiotics, surgery	Nervous system, energy, brain, growth, muscles, heart, digestion, and food metabolism, intestinal health, mouth, ears, appetite, blood building, circulation, learning	Stress, irritability, nervousness, depression, fatigue, diarrhea, constipation, indigestion, anemia, poor appetite
Alcohol, sugar, tobacco, caffeine	Health eyes, hair, skin and mouth, food metabolism, red blood and antibody formation, oxygenation of cells, growth	Cracks and sores at corners of mouth, sore tongue, athlete's foot, acne, oily face, poor growth, poor vision, nervousness, itching eyes, stress, indigestion, baldness

Nutrients	RDA/SDR Levels	Food Sources
B-3: niacin or niacinamide—most effective with B-complex, C, B-1, B-2, phosphorus	RDA 20 mg SDR 20-500 mg (Niacinamide form minimizes flushing of skin	Nutritional yeast, whole grains, rice, bran, prunes, apricots, citrus, nuts, cayenne, lean meat, fish, poultry, mushrooms, green vegetables, beans
B-5: pantothenic acid—most effective with B-complex, B-12, B-6, C, folic acid, biotin	RDA 10 mg SDR 40-100 mg	Whole grains, wheat germ, mushrooms, eggs, liver, salmon, nutritional yeast, molasses, legumes (beans & peas)
B-6: pyridoxine—most effective with B-complex, F, C, potassium, magnesium	RDA 2 mg SDR 10-60 mg	Whole wheat, brown rice, other whole grains, molasses, liver, bran of rice, wheat and corn, nutritional yeast, milk, egg yolk, fish, cabbage, beets, green leafy vegetables
B-12: cobalamin—most effective with B-complex, C, potassium, folic acid, calcium	RDA 6 mg SDR 20-100 mg	Cheese, fish, milk, cottage cheese, pork, liver, beef, eggs, soy tempeh, spirulina, kelp, pollen, comfrey (supplement is also necessary for strict vegetarians)

Appendix

Antagonists	Body Parts & Functions Aided	Deficiency Symptoms & Beneficial Uses
Stress, infection, sugar, caffeine, alcohol, antibiotics, trauma	Food metabolism (especially sugar, nervous system, digestion, adrenal glands, sex hormones, tongue, improves circulation	High blood pressure, poor circulation, cold extremities, leg cramps, migraine headaches, depression, nervousness, fatigue, pellagra, acne, skin eruptions, poor digestion, canker sores, halitosis (bad breath)
Stress, caffeine, alcohol, antibiotics, meat, insecticides	Adrenal glands (stress resistance), digestion, food metabolism, skin, nerves, growth, energy, convulsion, anti-body formation, vitamin utilization	Stress, weak adrenal glands, allergies, nervousness, duodenal ulcers, exhaustion, arthritis, dizziness, digestive disorders, graying hair, hair loss, hypoglycemia, retarded growth, premature aging, skin abnormalities
X-rays, caffeine, alcohol, tobacco, birth control pills	Nerves, blood, antibodies, muscles, skin, health, sodium-potassium balance, food metabolism and digestion, weight control, red blood cells	Stress, nervousness, depression, insomnia, irritability, dizziness, overweight, diuretics, high cholesterol, atherosclerosis, hardening of arteries, acne, hypoglycemia, anemia, nausea in pregnancy, bursitis
Laxatives, caffeine, alcohol, tobacco	Nervous system, helps iron build red blood, growth, appetite, food metabolism, cell longevity	Pernicious anemia, general weakness, fatigue, loss of appetite, nervousness, allergies, stress, shingles, nerve degeneration, overweight, walking & speaking difficulties

Appendix

NUTRIENTS	RDA/SDR LEVELS	FOOD SOURCES
Biotin: part of B-complex— most effective with B-complex, C, B-12, folic acid	RDA 300 mcg SDR 100-200 mcg	Eggs, liver, whole wheat, brown rice, other whole grains, nutritional yeast, lentils, sardines, poultry
Inositol: part of B-complex —most effective with B-complex, C, B-1, B-2, B-12, phosphorus, choline, linoleic acid	RDA 60 mg SDR 50-300 mg	Lecithin, whole grains, citrus, nutritional yeast, vegetables, liver, molasses, nuts, milk, meat, eggs, wheat germ
D (natural form): cholecalciferol— most effective with A, C, phosphorus, calcium, choline	RDA 400 IU SDR 400-800 IU	Sunshine, fish, liver oil, egg yolk, liver, salmon, tuna, herring, cod liver oil, (synthesized form of D is found in milk)
E: d-alpha tocopherol (not Dl-alpha)— most effective with B-complex, A, C, F, manganese, selenium	RDA 30 IU SDR 50-800 IU Older persons and those with heart problems should not begin with a high dosage	Whole grains, wheat germ oil, and cold-pressed vegetable oil, seeds, nuts, soybeans, eggs, organ meats, dark green vegetables

Appendix 165

ANTAGONISTS	BODY PARTS & FUNCTIONS AIDED	DEFICIENCY SYMPTOMS & BENEFICIAL USES
Oxidation, alcohol, caffeine, antibiotics, raw egg white	Food metabolism, hair and cell growth, B-complex utilization, fatty acid production, conversion of nucleic acids	Muscle pain, exhaustion, depression, hair loss, dry or graying hair, dermatitis, poor appetite
Sugar, caffeine, alcohol, antibiotics	Reduces cholesterol, metabolism of fats and cholesterol, atherosclerosis, constipation, overweight	Sleeplessness, eczema, hair loss, eye problems, high cholesterol, atherosclerosis, constipation, overweight
Mineral oil	Bone and teeth formation, calcium absorption, phosphorus assimilation, nerves, thyroid, blood clotting	Soft bones and teeth, bone disease, tooth decay, gum disease, nervousness, poor metabolism, muscular weakness, diarrhea, eczema, psoriasis, arthritis
Ultraviolet oxidation, rancid fat and oil, mineral oil, chlorine, birth control pills, air pollution, inorganic iron (ferrous sulphate and ferrous chloride)	Blood flow to heart, circulation, antioxidant (slows aging and preserves fats and oils, retards blood clotting, reproduction, cell oxygenation, prostate, blood and capillary maintenance, muscle and nerve maintenance, healthy hair and skin, lung protection	Heart disease, strokes, atherosclerosis, high cholesterol, calcium deposits, muscular dystrophy, enlarged prostate, impotence, sterility, menopausal and menstrual problems, miscarriage, cystitis, thrombosis, phlebitis, varicose veins

Nutrients	RDA/SDR Levels	Food Sources
Unsaturated fatty acids: most effective with E, A, D, C, phosphorus	RDA 2 tablespoons SDR 10% of total calories	Wheat germ and vegetable oils, seeds, cod liver oil
Choline: part of B-complex— most effective with B-complex, A, linoleic acid, inositol	RDA 60 mg SDR 50-250 mg	Eggs, wheat germ, legumes, liver, soybeans, lecithin, nutritional yeast
Folic acid: part of B-complex— most effective with B-complex, B-12, C, biotin, pantothenic acid	RDA 400 mcg SDR 400-2000 mcg	Green leafy vegetables, nutritional yeast, tuna, salmon, oysters, whole grains, mushrooms, liver, milk, nuts, dry beans
PABA: para-aminobenzoic acid— most effective with B-complex, C, folic acid	RDA 10 mg SDR 10-100 mg	Green vegetables, wheat germ, liver, nutritional yeast, molasses, milk, meat

Appendix 167

Antagonists	Body Parts & Functions Aided	Deficiency Symptoms & Beneficial Uses
Radiation, oxidation (air), mineral oil	Health of skin and hair, sex organs, glands, mucus membranes, growth, prevent cholesterol buildup, lubrication and resilience of skin	Dry skin disorders, eczema, psoriasis, acne, dry hair, dandruff, high cholesterol, heart disease, rheumatoid arthritis, gallstones, diarrhea, menopause
Sugar, alcohol, caffeine, insecticides	Hair, thymus gland, gall bladder and liver regulation, weight control, metabolism of fats, nerve transmission, healthy arteries, reduces cholesterol	High cholesterol, hardening of the arteries (atherosclerosis), high blood pressure, cirrhosis of liver, hair loss, stomach ulcers, gallstones, ringing in ears, dizziness, overweight
Stress, alcohol, caffeine, tobacco, streptomycin	Red blood cells, body growth and reproduction, protein metabolism, hydrochloric acid production, healthy, glands and liver	Anemia, B-12 deficiency, fatigue, slow growth, menstrual problems, birth defects, reproductive disorders, diarrhea, stress, graying hair, loss of hair
Caffeine, alcohol, sulfonamides	Skin, hair, intestines, protein, metabolism, muscles, hair color restoration, natural sunscreen	Fatigue (especially after muscle use), graying hair, dark skin spots, poor intestinal activity, folic acid production, anemia, headaches

Nutrients	RDA/SDR Levels	Food Sources
C: ascorbic acid— most effective with all vitamins, minerals and bioflavonoids	RDA 50-100 mg SDR 250-3000 mg Intake from 5000-15,000 mg may cause diarrhea in some individuals	Fresh fruit and vegetables, including alfalfa sprouts
K	SDR 30-100 mcg	Kelp, alfalfa, green vegetables, other green plants, eggs, milk, cauliflower, soy beans, polyunsaturated oil, yogurt
Bioflavonoids: rutin, hesperidin— most effective with C, calcium, magnesium	RDA 500 mg SDR 50-500 mg	Citrus, buckwheat, green pepper, black currants, cherries, grapes, onions, garlic, parsley, tomato

ANTAGONISTS	BODY PARTS & FUNCTIONS AIDED	DEFICIENCY SYMPTOMS & BENEFICIAL USES
Stress, alcohol, caffeine, tobacco, mercury, fever, overcooking, aspirin, cortisone, pasteurization, pollution, sulfonomides, perspiration	Teeth, gums, bones, blood and blood vessels, infection, resistance, collagen production, iron assimilation, wound healing, vitamin protection (anti-oxidant, aids longevity, adrenals	Susceptibility to infections (colds, viruses, flu, etc.), allergies, stress, anemia, blood vessel rupture, (hemorrhoids, bruising, varicose veins, nosebleeds) bleeding gums, dental cavities, atherosclerosis, cystitis, arthritis
Mineral oil, rancid fats, X-rays, antibiotics, aspirin	Bile absorption, growth, cell longevity, promotes blood coagulation, liver function	Hemorrhaging and prolonged bleeding, hemophilia, nosebleeds, prolonged menstruation, miscarriages and cellular disease
Stress, high fever, alcohol, tobacco, aspirin, excess salt, cortisone, air pollution	Blood vessel and capillary strength, resistance to infection, connective tissue, vitamin C utilization	Bruising, nosebleeds, hemorrhoids, varicose veins, duodenal ulcers, miscarriages, colds

MINERALS

Nutrients	RDA/SDR Levels	Food Sources
Calcium—most effective with A, C, D, F, magnesium, phosphorus, iron, manganese	RDA 800-1200 mg SDR 800-1500 mg	Dairy, dark green vegetables, sesame seeds, and sesame tahini, legumes, tofu, nuts, seaweed
Chromium	RDA 50-200 mcg SDR 100-300 mcg	Nutritional yeast, whole grains, clams, corn oil, liver, lean meat
Copper—most effective with zinc, cobalt, iron, C	RDA 2-3 mg SDR .5-2 mg	Seafood, seaweed, nuts, raisins, green leafy vegetables, soybeans, legumes, whole grains, liver
Iodine	RDA 150 mcg SDR 100-255 mcg	Wheat germ, fish, kelp tablets, seaweed, mushroom, garlic

ANTAGONISTS	BODY PARTS & FUNCTIONS AIDED	DEFICIENCY SYMPTOMS & BENEFICIAL USES
Stress and lack of exercise	Bones, teeth, heart rhythm, endurance, blood clotting, iron utilization, and relaxation of nerves	Sore muscles, backache, muscle cramps, premenstrual tension, menopause problems, brittle nails and bones, bone disease, nerve problems, insomnia, heart palpitations, arthritis, tooth and gum problems
Air pollution, sugar, metabolism	Blood sugar levels, increases effect of insulin, circulatory system, metabolism of glucose (energy), thyroid and adrenal glands	Glucose intolerance, hypoglycemia, diabetes, atherosclerosis
Excess zinc	Enzymes, elastin, red blood, hair and skin color, bone formation, iron absorption, healing process	Pernicious anemia, general weakness, skin sores, respiratory problems, retarded growth
None	Thyroid, metabolic rate, fat metabolism, energy production, hair, skin, nails, teeth, growth, speech, mental development	Goiter, hypothyroidism, hyperthyroidism, obesity, atherosclerosis, cold extremities, irritability, dry hair

Nutrients	RDA/SDR Levels	Food Sources
Iron—most effective with C, B-12, B-6, folic acid, copper, phosphorus, calcium, HCL acid	RDA 18 mg SDR 15-30 mg	Liver, wheat germ, oysters, molasses, green leafy vegetables, legumes, poultry, fish, eggs, dried fruit, whole grains
Magnesium—most effective with C, D, B-6, calcium, phosphorus, protein	RDA 400 mg SDR 300-500 mg	Dark green vegetables, whole grains, wheat germ, fish, seaweed, molasses, nuts, legumes, seeds
Manganese—most effective with B-1, E, calcium, phosphorus	RDA 2.5-5 mg SDR 5 mg	Whole grains, buckwheat, eggs, green vegetables, carrot, celery, beet, legumes, nuts, pineapples, liver, bran
Phosphorus—most effective with A, D, calcium, HCL acid, F, iron, protein	RDA 1000 mg SDR 50-150 mg	Lean meat, fish, poultry, eggs, whole grains, nuts, dairy, legumes, seeds, seaweed, green vegetables

Antagonists	Body Parts & Functions Aided	Deficiency Symptoms & Beneficial Uses
Coffee, bleeding, excess zinc and phosphorus, diarrhea	Hemoglobin, myoglobin, protein metabolism, energy, oxygen to muscle cells, stress, disease resistance, growth, health of skin, nails, teeth and bones	Anemia, blood loss, fatigue, pale skin, menstrual problems, brittle nails, breathing difficulties, constipation, colitis
Alcohol, diuretics, high cholesterol	Nerves, calcium and vitamin C absorption, bones, arteries, muscles, teeth, heart, memory, acid-alkaline balance, blood sugar metabolism (energy)	Calcium deposits, kidney stones, arteriosclerosis, heart problems, blood clots, nervousness, irritability, exhaustion, muscle twitches, confusion, convulsions, (epilepsy), tooth decay, soft bones (osteoporosis), stomach acid (as antacid)
Excess phosphorus and calcium	Enzyme activation, fat and carbohydrate metabolism, bones, sex hormones, growth, spleen, brain, pancreas, heart	Dizziness, diabetes (glucose intolerance), loss of muscular coordination, glandular disorders, hearing loss or noises, male impotence and sterility
Antacids, sugar, excess fats, aluminum, magnesium, iron	Bone and tooth formation, cell growth and repair, brain, nerve and muscle activity, vitamin utilization, energy, food metabolism, calcium and sugar metabolism, heart contractions	Bone disease, nervous disorders, stress, weakness, fatigue, tooth and gum disorders, stunted growth, weight problems, irregular breathing

Nutrients	RDA/SDR Levels	Food Sources
Potassium—most effective with B-6, sodium	RDA 1500 mg SDR 100-500 mg	Whole grains, bananas, milk, prunes, raisins, figs, seaweed, green vegetables, legumes, fish, seeds, potatoes
Selenium (bound to yeast)—most effective with vitamin E	RDA 50-200 mcg SDR 50-200 mcg Toxicity 500 mcg	Nutritional yeast, eggs, garlic, whole grains, broccoli, onions, tomato, tuna, seaweed, herring, seeds, mushrooms
Zinc—most effective with A, copper, calcium, phosphorus	RDA 15 mg SDR 20-50 mg	Liver, whole grains, eggs, mushrooms, nuts, bran, leafy vegetables, pumpkin and sunflower seeds, fish, nutritional yeast, soybeans
Sodium—most effective with vitamin D and potassium	RDA 1100 mg SDR none	Salt, dairy products, seafood and seaweed, meat, poultry, green vegetables
Chlorine—excess destroys vitamin E, intestinal flora	RDA 500 mg SDR none	Potassium chloride or table salts, seaweed, rye, oats, salt water fish

Appendix

Antagonists	Body Parts & Functions Aided	Deficiency Symptoms & Beneficial Uses
Diuretics, caffeine, alcohol, laxatives, stress, cortisone, excess salt and sugar, vomiting	Kidney functions, heartbeat, muscle contraction, skin, proper alkalinity, enzyme reactions, nerves, potassium-sodium balance	Irregular heartbeat, toxic kidneys, nervousness, insomnia, dry skin, acne, muscle damage, general weakness, high blood pressure
Mercury poisoning	Tissue elasticity, scalp, metabolism, growth, antioxidant, fertility, immune system, neutralizes carcinogens, pancreatic function	Premature aging, insomnia, inflexibility, dandruff, arteriosclerosis, impaired male sexual function
Lack of phosphorus, alcohol, excess calcium	Sex organs, brain, hair, prostate, skin, DNA-RNA synthesis, wound and burn healing, digestion and metabolism, B-complex utilization	Prostate problems, loss of taste, poor appetite, sterility, fatigue, retarded growth, diabetes, infertitlity, delayed sexual maturity
Chlorine, lack of potassium, diuretics	Normal cellular fluid level, osmotic cell pressure, proper muscle contraction, alkaline balance, blood, lymph	Weight loss, alkalosis, muscle cramps, dehydration, dry tongue Excess symptoms: high blood pressure, poor protein absorption, fluid retention (edema), thirst, insomnia, nervousness, irritability
	Protein digestion, liver cleansing, hydrochloric acid production, acid-alkaline balance, osmotic cell pressure, destroys bad bacteria & parasites in stomach	Hair and tooth loss, impaired digestion, poor muscle contraction